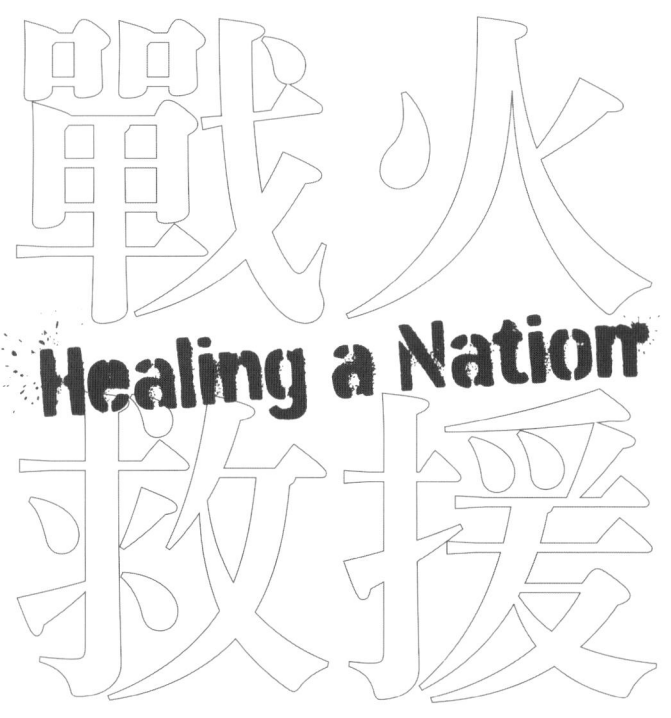

圖說二戰時期中美醫療合作
A Photographic History of
Sino-American Medical Collaboration During WWII

主編 / 楊善堯
翻譯 / 皮妤珊
審閱 / 陳榮彬
作者 / Sophia Hu（胡雪慧）、Catherine Liu（劉天悅）
Angelina Pi（皮妤姍）、Ellie Wang（王寶琪）

喆閎人文

目次
Contents

- 06 Editor's Words 主編序

- 10 Introduction
- 18 引言

- 36 Infrastructure, Transportation, and Communication
- 45 基礎建設、運輸、通訊

- 78 Operations and Advancements
- 88 醫療行動與進步

- 117 Working and Living Conditions
- 127 戰地工作與生活環境

- 160 Conclusion
- 163 結語

- 173 References 參考資料

主編序
Editor's Words

This book is a photography album that combines military history, archival images, historical humanities teaching, and international relations between the Republic of China (Taiwan) and the United States.

The origin of this series of historical photo books can be traced back to an international exchange activity. In June 2023, a group of Chinese-American high school students and their parents came to Taiwan under the leadership of Dr. Lin Hsiao-ting(林孝庭), the research fellow from the Hoover Institution of Stanford University. They visited the Presidential Palace, Academia Historica, National Revolutionary Martyrs' Shrine, Chiang Kai-shek Memorial Hall, the Palace Museum, the Grand Hotel, Fu Jen Catholic University, Longshan Temple, Bopiliao Historic Block, Daxi Old Street, and other places with strong "Republican, Chinese, and Taiwanese local culture" style. When they saw these scenic spots, they realized not only the historical and cultural significance behind these sites, but also their connections related to what they learned in the United States and their family backgrounds. This tour gives this group of high school students who came to Taiwan (Republic of China) for the first time a considerable cultural shock. During the visit, they constantly realized that the Republic of China is highly related to the United States where they grew up. This inspired their motivation and interest in exploring this period of history, which was the origin of this book.

Regarding the military cooperation between the Republic of China and the United States in the early twentieth century, it can be traced from the later stages of the War of Resistance against Japanese (1937-1945). When the Chinese government waged a full-scale and arduous warfare, the United States gave China considerable support, from civilian assistance to formal military aids. In the 1950s, while economy of Taiwan gained highly development with the U.S. aids, the military cooperation between the Republic of China and the United States is also a vital part of the Cold War history. The subject of this book, "battlefield medical rescue", is an important part of Sino-American military cooperation.

The four authors of this book, Sophia Hu(胡雪慧), Catherine Liu(劉天悅), Angelina Pi(皮妤姍), and Ellie Wang(王寶琪), use historical photos and archives collected by the U.S. National Archives, and the Zhe Hong Humanities Studio(喆閎人文工作室) to present the subject clearly and richly through chronological arrangement. The impact of visual images is far greater than the feelings that words bring to readers. I hope the publication of this photo album, interpretation of the historical archives by four high school students, will attract more people's attention to this period of history, and help readers understand that historical archives are not only for scholars, even high school students can use them to complete a project.

Yang, Shan-Yao
2025.5.27

這本書是一本結合軍事歷史、檔案影像、歷史人文教學、中華民國（臺灣）與美國國際關係的攝影冊。

　　這個系列歷史照片書籍的源起，要從一次的國際交流活動談起。2023 年 6 月，一群美籍華裔高中生與家長，在史丹佛大學胡佛研究所林孝庭研究員的帶領下來到了臺灣，在總統府、國史館、忠烈祠、中正紀念堂、故宮博物院、圓山飯店、輔仁大學、龍山寺、剝皮寮、大溪老街等地方進行了參訪與交流，這些帶有濃厚「民國風、中華文化、臺灣在地文化」風格的景點，以及這些景點帶來的實體視覺與景點背後所隱含的歷史文化意義，都與他們從小在美國所學以及家庭文化有所關聯，給了這群第一次來到臺灣（中華民國）的高中生們相當大的文化衝擊。在參訪的過程中，他們不斷地發現到一個問題：「中華民國跟他們所生長的美國有著高度關聯性」，這引起了他們去探索這段歷史過往的動機與興趣，也是這本書誕生的緣起。

　　有關中華民國與美國在二十世紀的軍事往來，可從抗日戰爭的中後期開始談起。在中華民國政府進行全面性的艱苦戰爭時，美國從民間援助到正式軍援，給了當時中華民國政府相當大的支持，到了 1950 年代後，在美援支持下臺灣快速的全面復甦，尤其在軍事上的援助，更是冷戰時代下中華民國與美國的重要連結。這本書所講述的「戰地醫療救護」主題，正好是串聯起這段中華民國與美國友好過往的重要歷史。

　　Sophia Hu（胡雪慧）、Catherine Liu（劉天悅）、Angelina Pi（皮妤姍）、Ellie Wang（王寶琪）四位作者利用美國國家檔案館與喆閎人文工作室所典藏的歷史照片與檔案，透過照片解讀與時序排列，清楚且豐富的呈現出「戰地醫療救護」這個主題。視覺影像的渲染力與感受力遠大於單純文字給讀者帶來的感受，希望這本攝影冊的面世，透過作者解讀歷史檔案的過程，能引起更多人對於這段歷史的注意，以及讓歷史人文融入應用實作有更多的成果展現。

楊善堯

民國一一四年五月廿七日

INTRODUCTION

The International Medical Relief Corps (IMRC) was formed in the late 1930s, driven by international leftist networks of medical professionals who had gained wartime experience during the Spanish Civil War from 1936 to 1939. After the Republican defeat in Spain, many of these doctors were displaced and sought new opportunities to aid anti-fascist causes.

As China fought Japan in the Second Sino-Japanese War from 1937 to 1945, the IMRC was created to send volunteer doctors and medical supplies to support the Chinese war effort. The corps provided mobile medical units, field hospitals, and training for Chinese medical staff, particularly in areas controlled by Communist forces. The IMRC's work significantly impacted medical practices in China, and its members are still celebrated there for their contributions.

The Second Sino-Japanese War

Japan's imperialistic ambitions and the unresolved tensions of power dynamics between Japan and China came to a front on July 7, 1937, when the Marco Polo Bridge Incident escalated into a full-scale war between Japan and China. As Japanese forces pushed into Chinese territories, the damage inflicted on civilian populations called for the urgent need for humanitarian assistance. Atrocities such as the Nanjing Massacre of 1937 stood out due to their brutality and the sheer scale of casualties.

At the center of China's resistance to Japanese aggression were two major political forces: the Guomindang Nationalist Party and the Chinese Communist Party. The Guomindang, under the leadership of Chiang Kai-shek, embodied a nationalist and capitalist vision for a modern China, while the Chinese Communist Party, led by Mao Zedong, promoted a radically different communist and socialist future. Despite their ideological differences and long-standing rivalry, their shared suffering during the war pushed the two opposing parties into an uneasy alliance. Their combined efforts, although filled with internal tensions, were essential to creating a national resistance against the encroaching Japanese forces.

Sino-American Collaboration

Even though the United States had initially claimed neutrality, the nation was soon drawn into war following a series of provocative attacks from the Japanese. Its breaking point, the attack on Pearl Harbor on December 7, 1941, outraged Americans and served as a catalyst compelling the public to shift away from its isolationist sentiment. Although World War II had started years before, in 1939, the United States declared war against Japan on December 8, 1941, formally entering the war.

As the war intensified, the United States found itself increasingly intertwined with the Sino-Japanese conflict. American policymakers and military strategists soon began to recognize that the outcome of the Sino-Japanese War would affect the broader outcomes of World War II; if Japan were to successfully imperialize China and the rest of Asia, it would cause more harm for the Allied Powers. As a result, the United States adopted a "the enemy of my enemy is my friend" mindset and began to view support for China as not only a strategic necessity but also a moral imperative. The Lend-Lease Act, passed on March 11, 1941, enabled the United States to provide aid to China, including military supplies and medical resources. This involvement contributed to the birth of resistance efforts in America that were created with the goal of assisting China.

United States Support

By 1938, the ongoing invasion by the Imperial Japanese Army had forced both the Chinese Communist Party and the Guomindang Nationalist Party into retreat. Pushed into the western interior of China, these rivalling parties continued resisting through guerilla campaigns. However, their lack of cooperation resulted in strategic inefficiencies and unnecessary losses. The Chinese Army Medical Administration, already struggling with limited resources, was overwhelmed by the rapidly increasing numbers of casualties from both direct Japanese attacks and the reckless guerilla warfare. The severe shortage of trained medical personnel and supplies further exacerbated the suffering of both soldiers and civilians.

Recognizing the need for organized humanitarian assistance, efforts to provide aid began to intensify. One of the most notable initiatives was the establishment of the Chinese Red Cross Medical Relief Corps, which was part of a broader response to the shared devastation wrought by aggressive military campaigns internationally by Germany and Japan. Leading the new Corps was Dr. Robert Lin, also known as Lin Kesheng (Lín Kěshèng), who was a highly respected investigator, clinician, and professor at the Beijing Union Medical College. Charismatic and deeply patriotic, Dr. Robert Lin was widely admired by both Chinese politicians and common citizens. Under his leadership, the Chinese Red Cross Medical Relief Corps gained importance as they provided the Emergency Medical Services Training School and the first use of a blood bank. This collective effort trained over 15000 medical personnel, significantly bolstering emergency medical services.

Following the creation of the Chinese Red Cross, China began to receive backing from various international organizations and American Chinese communities. The China Aid Council, founded in New York City in 1937, was composed of Chinese emigrants and American supporters. The organization focused on fundraising efforts to purchase vital medical equipment and supplies for refugees and wounded soldiers, channeling financial and material aid to the regions of China that were especially affected by the war.

The established by Chinese Americans in 1937, played another critical role in bridging the gap between the Chinese Red Cross and international donors. Through ABMAC, shipments of medical supplies reached the Red Cross Society of the Republic of China, ensuring that hospitals and field clinics remained operational despite overwhelming demand.

The American Red Cross, a well-established humanitarian organization founded after the American Civil War, extended its reach to China as part of its global relief efforts. Although they were originally focused on the United States and Europe, the American Red Cross later turned to assist China as well. In addition to sending resources overseas, the organization also directly mobilized volunteers, deployed teams of medical personnel to train local staff, distributed emergency supplies, and established mobile clinics in the besieged regions. Their presence not only provided immediate medical care but also helped improve the overall infrastructure of China's medical services during wartime.

United China Relief was founded in 1941 in New York City with a distinct mission to raise at least five million dollars for China's humanitarian relief. The organization garnered support from influential figures, including actress Anna May Wong, hosted fundraising events, performances, and publication campaigns that were launched to solicit donations. Through booklets, pamphlets, and public speeches, United China Relief was able to spread awareness of the effects of the war, which further rallied widespread support for Chinese people.

Origins of the IMRC

The Spanish Civil War from 1936 to 1939 and the Second Sino-Japanese War from 1937 to 1945 were connected through a network of international leftist solidarity, as doctors from around the world responded to the anti-fascist cause. During the Spanish Civil War, many foreign doctors volunteered to aid the Republican—or anti-fascist—side, particularly through the International Brigades and medical organizations like the British Medical Aid Unit. These doctors gained invaluable experience treating war injuries in difficult conditions and working under pressure with limited resources.

However, after the Republicans' defeat in 1939, Francisco Franco's Nationalist forces established a fascist dictatorship and many of these doctors, most of whom were leftists, socialists, communists, or simply anti-fascist, were displaced. With the rise of right-wing governments in Europe and North America, particularly those governments hostile toward individuals with communist ties, many doctors found it difficult to secure jobs or visas. Some doctors fled to France or other countries, seeking asylums or refuge from persecution.

Foreign Doctors

As World War II broke out in 1939, Europe's focus shifted toward their own survival, leaving many of the displaced doctors from the Spanish Civil War without guidance. However, some doctors, particularly those with communist sympathies, saw China's war against Japan as another front in the global battle against fascism and imperialism. Despite their fears, they were once again motivated to continue to fight. British nurse Patience Darton wrote about the dilemma many Spanish doctors faced, lamenting that They wanted to go to China, because at least it was somewhere to be—they didn't particularly want to leave Europe, but they wanted to go on being somebody in something.

Many doctors in exile, though still hesitant, found inspiration in Edgar Snow's 1937 book, *Red Star Over China* which introduced them to the ideas of Mao Zedong and the Chinese Communist Party, further encouraging them to consider heading to China. The Communist International (Comintern), which was led by the Soviet Union, helped organize the import of Russian doctors into China, further cementing the connection between the Spanish Civil War and the growing international medical effort to assist China.

Among the most famous foreign volunteers was Dr. Henry Norman Bethune or Bai Qiu'en (Bái Qiú'ēn), a Canadian thoracic surgeon and member of the Communist Party of Canada. Dr. Norman Bethune had already served as a frontline trauma surgeon in Spain, where he developed the first mobile blood-transfusion service for battlefield operations. In 1938, his medical innovations and dedication to anti-fascist causes led him to China, where he worked under the leadership of Mao Zedong bringing modern medical practices to rural areas and supporting the Chinese Communist forces. His contributions were critical, and he treated sick villagers and soldiers alike, quickly becoming highly respected by the Chinese people. Tragically, Dr. Norman Bethune died from blood poisoning after accidentally cutting his finger while operating on wounded Chinese soldiers. He was deeply mourned, and Mao Zedong wrote a eulogy, "In Memory of Norman Bethune," dedicated to him. Today, Dr. Norman Bethune's story is still part of the Chinese school curriculum, and his work remains celebrated in China.

Another notable foreign volunteer was Dr. Adele Cohn or Ke'en (Kē'ēn), a strong-willed North American pulmonologist specializing in tuberculosis, a disease often referred to as "the white death" due to its high mortality rate. Despite the risks and opposition from an isolationist America, Dr. Adele Cohn volunteered to help in China for a year. The American Bureau of Medical Aid and the Chinese Red Cross sponsored her, and she went on to teach Chinese doctors how to treat tuberculosis. Initially, Dr. Robert Lin, who preferred excluding women from the medical corps, was tentative in accepting her. However, he overlooked his usual standards as Dr. Adele Cohn's qualifications, especially her expertise in tuberculosis, made her more than competent, even if she did not meet the gender or age requirements. Later, he began accepting more female physicians who did not meet his age and gender requirements due to their qualifications.

Also contributing to the medical efforts in China was Dr. Dwarakanath Shantaram Kotnis or Ke Dihua (Kē Dìhuá). Dr. Dwarakanath Kotnis went to China in 1938, where he joined the Eighth Route Army led by Mao Zedong. In one case, he treated more than eight hundred wounded soldiers during a particularly brutal battle in 1940 despite the immense stress and shortages of medical supplies. He worked tirelessly, often operating for 72 hours straight without sleep. Dr. Dwarakanath Kotnis was appointed Director of the Bethune International Peace Hospital after Dr. Norman Bethune's death, becoming a long-standing symbol of Sino-Indian friendship. Unfortunately, Dr. Dwarakanath Kotnis's health deteriorated due to the harsh conditions, and he died in 1942 from a series of epileptic seizures. His death was deeply mourned by Mao Zedong, and he is now commemorated with statues and memorials across China.

Many European Jewish doctors also joined the International Medical Relief Corps, including Heinrich Kohn, who changed his name to "Carner" Kent or Kende (Kěndé), and Wladyslaw Jungermann, who changed his name to "Wolf" Jungery or Rong Geman (Róng Gémàn). Others include George Schön/György Somogyi or Shen'en (Shěn'ēn) and Iacod Kranzdorf/Bucur Clejan or Ke Rangdao (KēRàngdào). After fleeing the pervasive anti-Semitism in Europe, these doctors changed their names and moved to China to escape persecution and contribute their expertise to the Chinese cause.

Eventually, the devastating consequences of World War II demonstrated to the Allied Powers that international collaboration not only gave them a strategic advantage but was also a moral necessity. Following the Spanish Civil War, the development of the International Medical Relief Corps became an essential part of the medical aid effort in China, organized by both the Soviet Union and international leftist networks. The doctors who joined the cause brought much-needed expertise to the frontlines, providing care to soldiers and civilians alike. Their sacrifices, both personal and professional, helped shape China's resistance against Japan and left a lasting legacy in the country's history.

引言

國際醫療救護隊（International Medical Relief Corps，簡稱 IMRC）成立於 1930 年代末期，由一群來自國際左翼組織的醫療專業人士組成，他們曾在 1936 至 1939 年的西班牙內戰中積累豐富戰地救援經驗。西班牙共和國政府敗北後，這些醫生流離失所，並尋找新的機會來支持反法西斯的志業。國際醫療救護隊創辦時，中國的抗日戰爭（1937 至 1945 年）剛好也在如火如荼進行中，於是該組織便派遣醫生來華進行志願服務，並給予醫療物資援助。他們組織了流動醫療隊、野戰醫院，並對中國醫療人員進行訓練，尤其是在共軍控制的地區。國際醫療救護隊的行動對中國醫療產生了深遠影響，其成員至今仍因其貢獻而在中國備受讚譽。

抗日戰爭

　　由於日本充滿帝國主義野心，中日關係始終處於緊張局勢，未能化解，最終在 1937 年 7 月 7 日因為盧溝橋事變導致中日戰爭全面爆發。隨著日軍入侵中國領土，平民深受戰火摧殘使人道救援的需求變得刻不容緩。眾多暴行中，以 1937 年的南京大屠殺尤為駭人，日軍種種慘無人道的暴行導致中國軍民傷亡慘重。

　　當時對抗日本侵略的主要是中國國內的兩股政治勢力：中國國民黨與中國共產黨。國民黨在蔣中正的領導下，是民族主義與資本主義現代化願景的代表，而毛澤東領導的中共則試圖推動與上述願景截然不同的共產主義與社會主義未來。儘管雙方在意識形態上存在巨大分歧，且長期相互對立，但戰爭中的共同苦難迫使這兩個敵對陣營勉強進行所謂「第二次國共合作」。此一合作關係雖充滿內部矛盾，卻是組織全國抵抗日軍入侵的關鍵力量。

中美合作

　　儘管美國最初聲稱中立，但在日本發動一連串充滿挑釁意味的攻擊後，終究被迫參戰。此一發展的轉折點是 1941 年 12 月 7 日的珍珠港事變，日軍的攻擊行動激起美國民眾的怒火，促使輿論轉變立場，摒棄孤立主義。儘管第二次世界大戰早在 1939 年便已爆發，美國直到 1941 年 12 月 8 日才對日宣戰，正式參與二戰。

隨著戰爭加劇，美國與中日戰爭的關係也日益緊密。美國的決策者與軍事戰略家很快意識到，中日戰爭的結果將影響整個二戰的局勢：若日本成功將中國及整個亞洲納入其帝國版圖，將對同盟國造成嚴重的威脅。因此，這種「敵人的敵人就是朋友」的思維促使美國改變心態，開始認為對華援助不只是戰略上的必要，更是道義上的責任。1941 年 3 月 11 日通過的《租借法案》使美國能夠向中國提供援助，包括軍事物資與醫療資源。這一介入行動也促使美國境內誕生了旨在支援中國的抗戰援助運動。

美援

到了 1938 年，日軍的持續侵略迫使中國共產黨與國民黨雙雙往後方撤退。在被迫退往中國西部內陸後，這兩股敵對勢力分別以游擊戰的方式抵抗日軍。由於兩黨缺乏協作，造成戰略成效不佳以及眾多不必要的損失。軍醫署（隸屬於國民政府軍事委員會軍政部）原本就資源匱乏，日軍的長驅直入和游擊戰造成傷亡人數急遽增加，更是使其不堪重負。嚴重缺少物資與醫療人員則加重了士兵與平民的苦難程度。

各界意識到中國需要有組織的人道援助，加速展開救援工作。為回應德國、日本在全球發動侵略行動帶來的大量災難，最重要的行動之一便是成立中國紅十字會救護總隊，總隊長由北京協和醫學院林可勝教授擔任，他是一位備受尊敬的學者與臨床醫生。渾身散發人格魅力的林博士是中國政界與民眾都敬仰的愛國人士。在他的領導下，紅十字會救護總隊發揮了舉足輕重的作用，包括設立戰時衛生人員訓練所，以及率先使用血庫技術。這次團結的努力成果共培訓超過 15,000 名醫療人員，大幅提升了戰時急救醫療服務的能力。

在中國紅十字會成立後，中國開始獲得來自各國際組織及美籍華人團體的支持。1937 年，由華人移民與美國親華人士組成的中國援助委員會（China Aid Council）在紐約成立。該組織專注於籌款購買必要的醫療設備與物資，用於援助難民與傷兵，並將經費與物資輸送至受戰火波及最為慘烈的中國地區。

1937年，由美籍華人成立的「美國醫藥助華會」（American Bureau of Medical Aid for China，簡稱 ABMAC）在銜接中國紅十字會與國際捐助者之間發揮了關鍵作用。該會協助將大批醫療物資送往中華民國紅十字會，以確保各地醫院與野戰醫院在需求激增的情況下仍能持續運作。

美國紅十字會（American Red Cross）是歷史悠久的人道救援組織，成立於美國內戰後，始終致力於全球救援行動。即便最初僅專注於對美國與歐洲的援助，美國紅十字會後來也將目光轉向中國。除了透過海運寄送救援物資給中國以外，該組織還直接動員志工，派遣醫療隊伍培訓當地人員，分發緊急物資，並在被圍困的地區設立流動診所。他們的援助不僅提供了即時的醫療救護，也在戰時大幅改善了中國的醫療基礎設施。

1941年，美國援華聯合會（United China Relief）在紐約成立，並以籌集至少五百萬美元的人道援助資金為目標。該組織獲得了許多知名人士的支持，包括華裔女演員黃柳霜，並透過舉辦募款活動、表演與出版宣傳等方式募集捐款。透過小冊子、宣傳單與公開演講，美國援華聯合會成功喚起外界對戰爭影響的關注，進一步凝聚了社會各界對中國人民的廣泛支持。

國際醫療救護隊的緣起

在西班牙內戰（1936至1939年）和抗日戰爭（1937至1945年）期間，來自世界各地的醫生透過國際左翼組織緊密合作，紛紛響應反法西斯的號召。西班牙內戰時，許多外國醫生自願支援共和派（即反法西斯陣營），尤其是透過國際縱隊（International Brigades）及英國醫療援助隊（British Medical Aid Unit）等組織，投入戰地救援工作。這些醫生在惡劣環境中治療戰傷，並在資源有限的情況下承受高壓工作，從而獲得了極為寶貴的實戰經驗。

然而,由於共和派於 1939 年戰敗,佛朗哥將軍領導的國民軍建立了法西斯獨裁政權,許多醫生因此流離失所。其中大多數人是左翼分子、社會主義者、共產主義者,或單純只是反法西斯人士。當時,右翼政府在歐洲與北美地區崛起,這些政府尤其敵視共產黨的相關人士,許多醫生因此難以獲得工作機會或簽證。一部分人選擇逃往法國或其他國家尋求庇護,以躲避政治迫害。

外籍醫生

隨著 1939 年第二次世界大戰爆發,歐洲各國轉而關注自身的生存問題,但也導致許多因西班牙內戰而流離失所的醫生陷入困境,不知該何去何從。然而,其中一群支持共產主義的醫生,將中國對日抗戰視為全球反法西斯與反帝國主義戰爭的另一條戰線。儘管對戰爭充滿恐懼,他們仍再次鼓起勇氣,選擇繼續奮鬥。英國護士佩申斯・達頓(Patience Darton)曾記錄許多西班牙醫生所面臨的兩難處境,她感慨道:「他們想去中國,因為那至少是一個能前往的地方——他們其實並不想離開歐洲,但他們希望能在某個地方有所作為。」

許多流亡的醫生雖仍心存猶豫,卻透過美國記者埃德加・斯諾(Edgar Snow)的著作《紅星照耀中國》(*Red Star Over China*,1937 年出版)受到啟發。這本書讓他們接觸到毛澤東與中共的理念,進一步促使他們考慮前往中國。由蘇聯主導的共產國際(Comintern)也協助安排俄國醫生進入中國,使西班牙內戰與國際對華醫療援助行動的關係更加緊密。

最著名的外國醫療志工之一是加拿大胸腔外科醫生白求恩(Henry Norman Bethune),他同時也是個加共黨員。白求恩曾在西班牙戰場擔任前線外科醫生,並在那裡創立了世界上第一支戰地流動輸血隊,為前線傷員提供即時的輸血服務。1938 年,堅決進行醫療創新堅定同時想對反法西斯志業有所貢獻的白求恩來到中國,在毛澤東的領導下,將現代醫療技術引入農村地區,並支援中國共產黨部隊。他的貢獻極為關鍵,不僅救治傷病共軍成員，也為鄉村百姓提供醫療服務，很快便贏得了中國人民的深厚敬重。不幸的是，白求恩在為受傷的中國軍人動手術時不慎割傷手指，因感染丹毒而引發敗血症後離世。他的逝世引發深切哀悼，毛澤東特別撰寫了悼詞〈紀念白求恩〉，以表對他的敬意。時至今日，白求恩的事蹟仍被納入中國的學校課程，他的貢獻在中國依然備受敬仰。

另一位著名的外國志工是美國肺病學專家科恩醫師（Adele Cohn）。她是一位意志堅定的結核病專家——這種疾病因高死亡率而有「白死病」之稱。當時美國奉行孤立主義，科恩醫師不過各種風險與反對聲音，毅然前往中國擔任醫療志工，為期一年。她的中國之行由美國醫藥助華會與中國紅十字會共同贊助，並在中國指導當地醫生如何治療結核病。最初，林可勝醫生對於是否接納她猶豫不決，因為他不希望紅十字會的醫療隊裡有女性成員。然而，科恩醫師卓越的專業能力——尤其是在結核病領域的專長，使她獲得破格錄取，即便她未符合既定的性別與年齡標準。此後，林可勝開始接受更多資歷足夠優秀的女性醫生，即使她們不符合他原訂的標準。

另一位對於中國醫療援助有所貢獻的外國醫生是柯棣華（Dwarakanath Shantaram Kotnis）。1938年，柯棣華來到中國加入毛澤東領導的八路軍。在1940年的一場極為慘烈的戰役中，儘管面臨著巨大壓力與醫療資源短缺，他仍奮力救治了800多名傷兵。柯棣華不知疲倦地工作，經常連續手術72小時不眠不休。在白求恩去世後，中共任命他接任「白求恩國際和平醫院」[1]的院長職務，他也成為中印友誼的象徵。然而，由於工作環境的條件不佳，他的健康逐漸惡化，最終於1942年因癲癇發作不幸去世。他的離世令毛澤東深感哀痛，如今，中國各地都為他豎立了雕像與紀念碑，以緬懷他的貢獻。

許多來自歐洲的猶太醫生也加入了國際醫療救護隊，其中包括海因里希·科恩（Heinrich Kohn，後改名為 "Carner" Kent，漢名肯德），以及瓦迪斯瓦夫·容格曼（Wladyslaw Jungermann，後改名為 "Wolf"

---

1 後來的正式名稱為「中國人民解放軍聯勤保障部隊第九八〇醫院」。

Jungery，漢名戎格曼）。其他成員還包括喬治・舍恩（George Schön，又名 György Somogyi，漢名沈恩），以及伊阿科德・克蘭茨多夫（Iacod Kranzdorf，又名 Bucur Clejan，漢名柯讓道）。由於當時歐洲的反猶太主義氛圍猖獗，他們改名換姓，遠赴中國，不僅是為了躲避迫害，更為了將自身的專業知識貢獻於中國的戰時醫療事業。

最終，第二次世界大戰的毀滅性後果讓同盟國認識到，國際合作不僅能帶來戰略優勢，更是一種道義上的責任。在西班牙內戰之後，國際醫療救護隊逐漸發展成援助中國醫療的重要力量，這一組織由蘇聯與國際左翼組織共同推動。參與這場醫療救援的醫生們將寶貴的專業知識帶到了前線，為傷兵與平民提供救治。他們在個人與職業上的犧牲，不僅強化了中國對抗日本的抵抗力量，也在中國歷史上留下了深遠的影響。

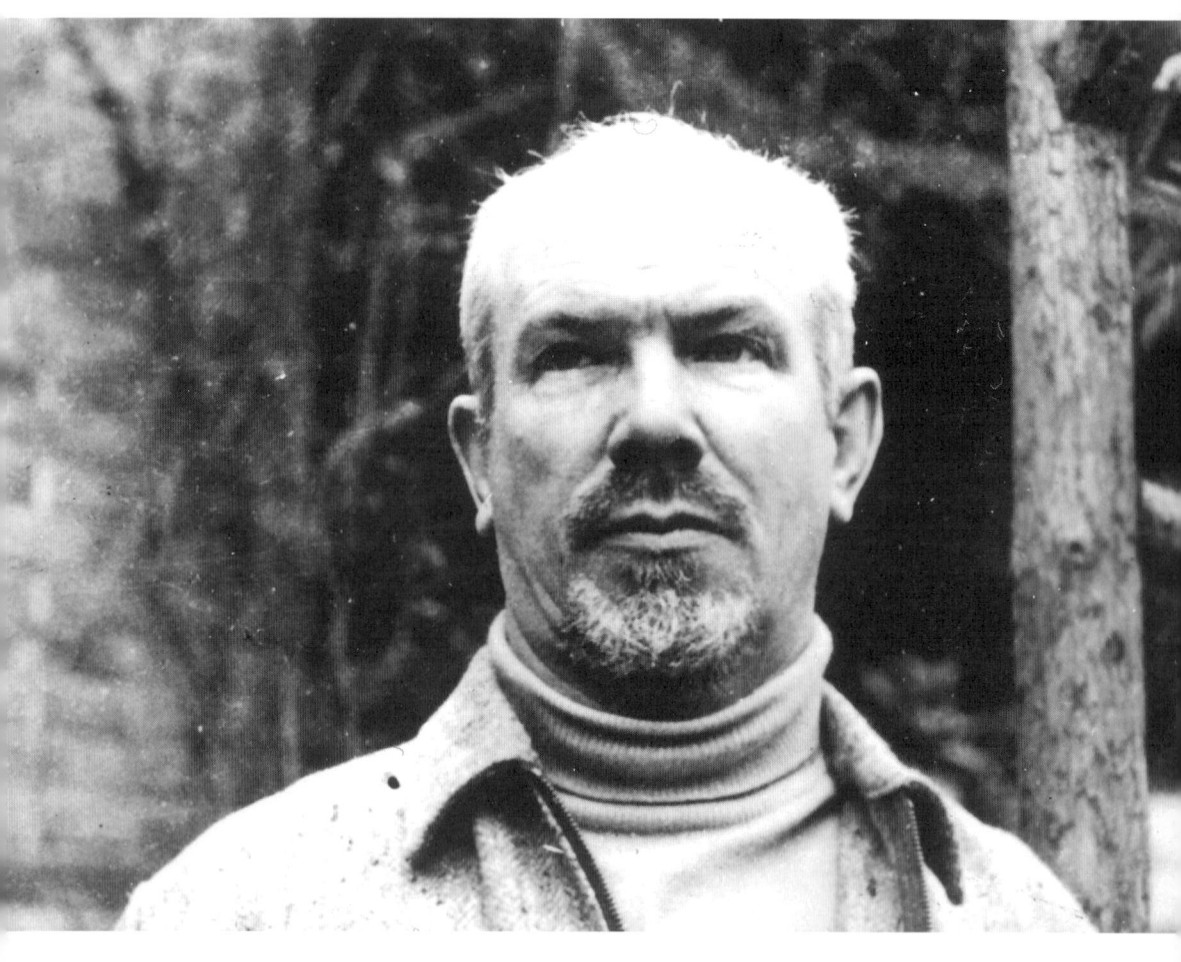

Dr. Henry Bethune was the founder of the International Peace Hospitals in China. He arrived in China in 1938, instructing and teaching his Chinese colleagues about surgery.

白求恩醫生是中國國際和平醫院的創辦人,他在 1938 年抵達中國,向中國同僚指導並教授外科手術技術。

Date of Photo 時間:不詳 N/A
Credits 來源:美國國家檔案館 Photo Courtesy of National Archives

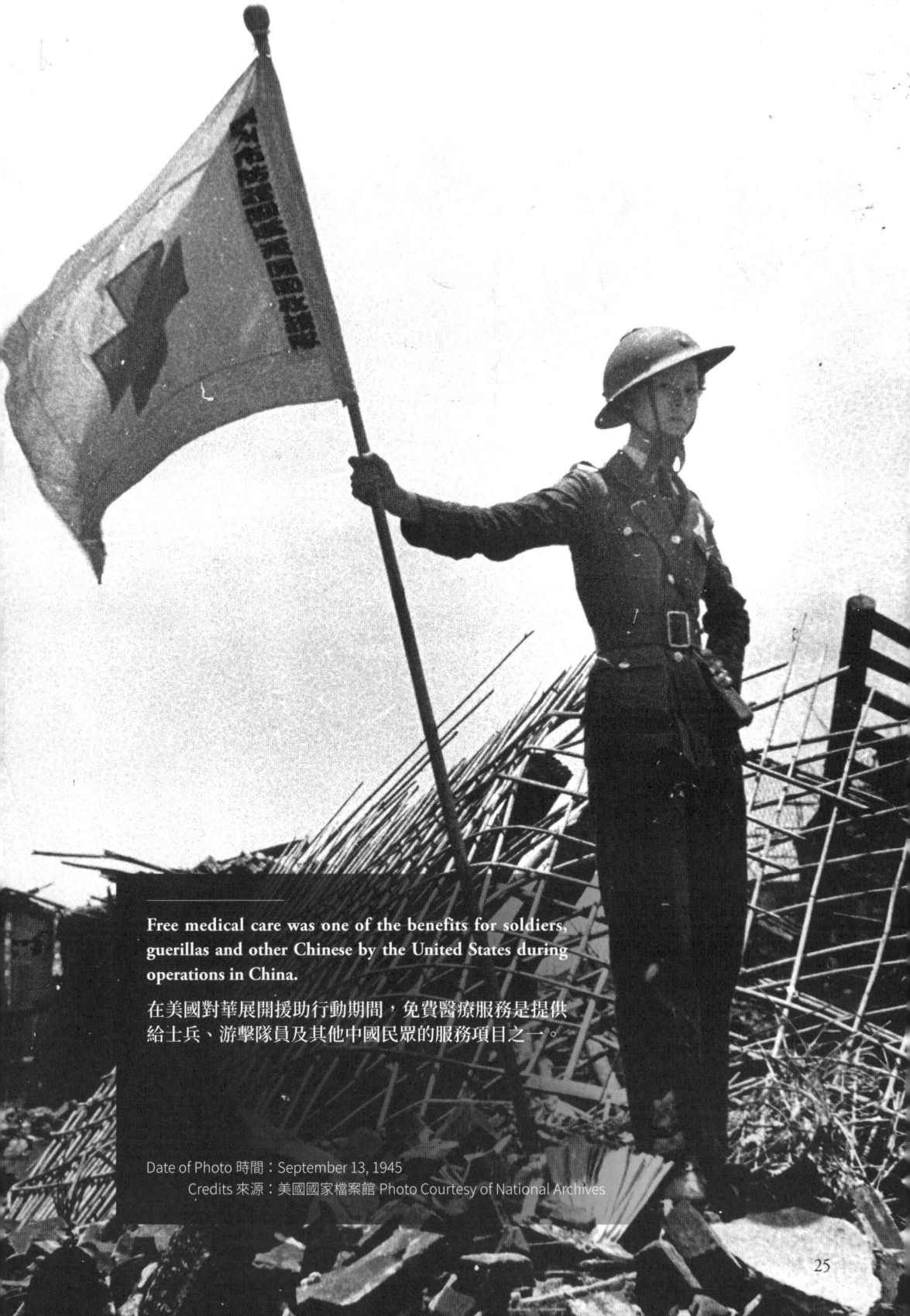

Free medical care was one of the benefits for soldiers, guerillas and other Chinese by the United States during operations in China.

在美國對華展開援助行動期間,免費醫療服務是提供給士兵、游擊隊員及其他中國民眾的服務項目之一。

Date of Photo 時間:September 13, 1945
Credits 來源:美國國家檔案館 Photo Courtesy of National Archives

Lieutenant Colonel Randle J. Brady performs a medical check-up on a Chinese soldier in Luliang, China.

陸軍中校蘭德・布雷迪在山西省呂梁為一名中國士兵看診。

Date of Photo 時間：March 11, 1945
Credits 來源：美國國家檔案館 Photo Courtesy of National Archives

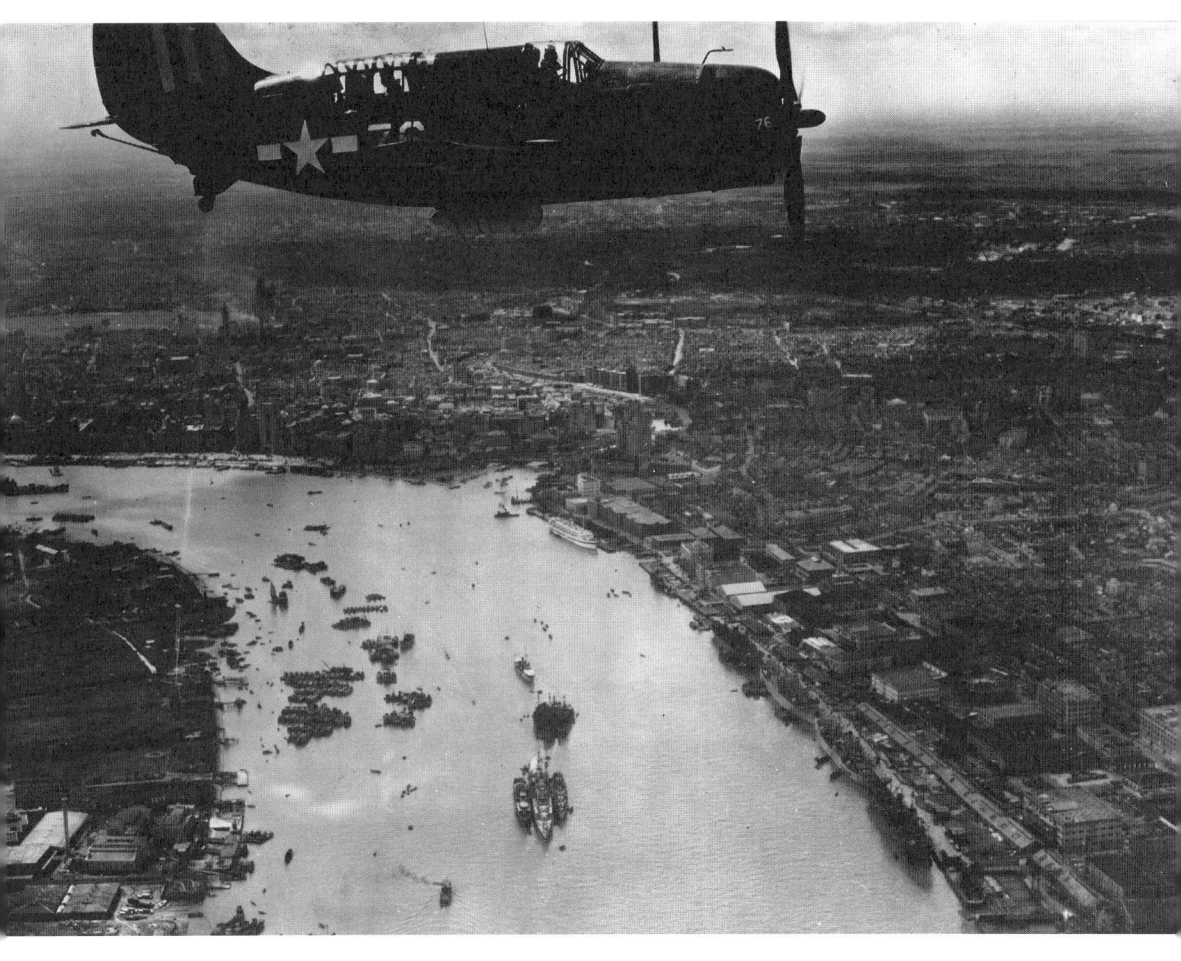

United States air ambulances were airplanes and helicopters that transport wounded soldiers from war zones to hospitals.

美國空中救護隊使用飛機與直升機,將戰場上的傷兵運送至醫院進行救治。

Date of Photo 時間:September 28, 1945
Credits 來源:美國國家檔案館 Photo Courtesy of National Archives

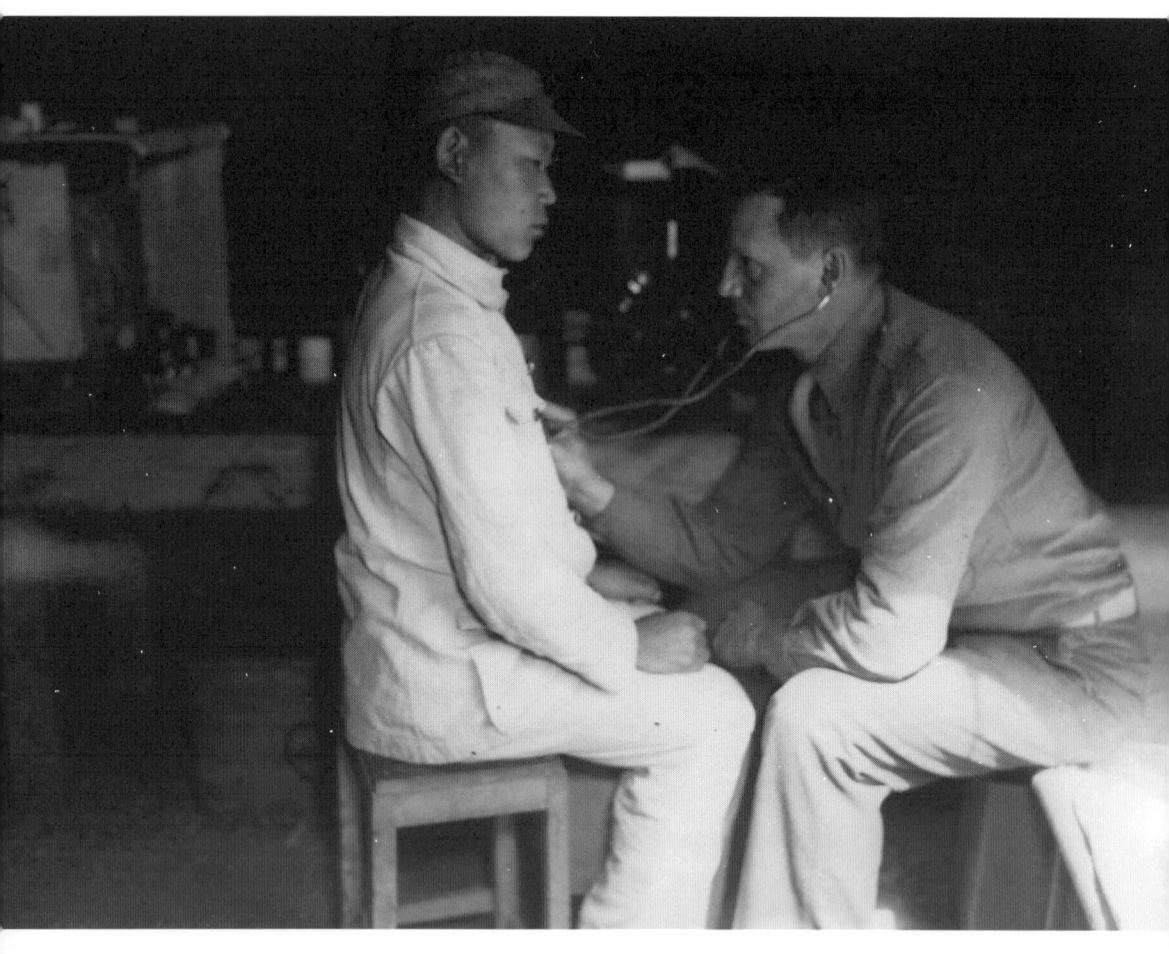

Lieutenant Colonel Randle J. Brady performs a medical check-up on a Chinese soldier in Luliang, China.

陸軍中校蘭德・布雷迪在山西省呂梁為一名中國士兵看診。

Date of Photo 時間：March 11, 1945
Credits 來源：美國國家檔案館 Photo Courtesy of National Archives

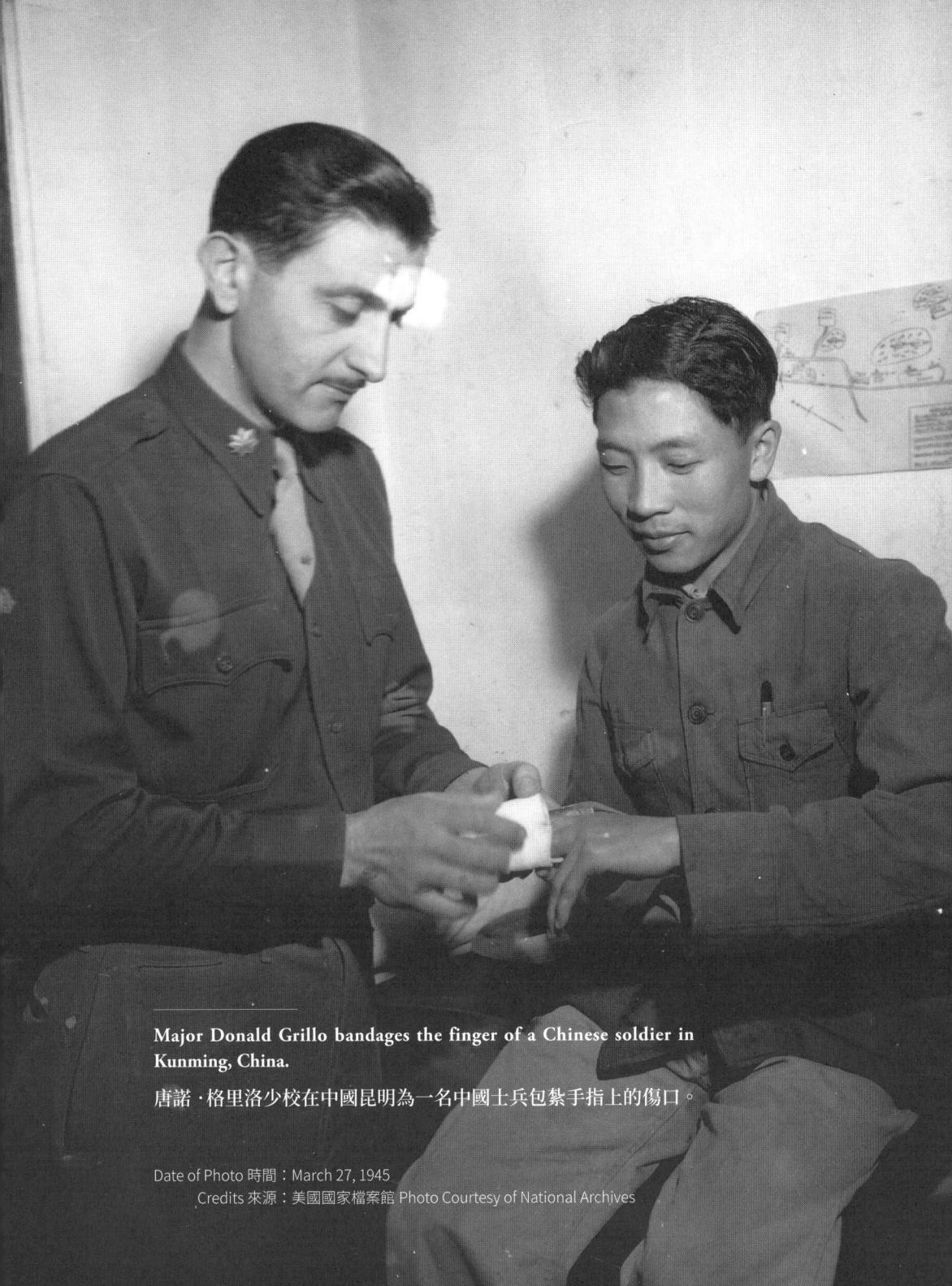

Major Donald Grillo bandages the finger of a Chinese soldier in Kunming, China.

唐諾‧格里洛少校在中國昆明為一名中國士兵包紮手指上的傷口。

Date of Photo 時間：March 27, 1945
Credits 來源：美國國家檔案館 Photo Courtesy of National Archives

Sergeant Arthur Bonko, an American aerial gunner of the 14th Air Force, recieved first aid after courageously destroying seven Japanese Army planes.

來華參與對日抗戰的美國第十四航空隊飛機炮手亞瑟・邦科英勇擊落七架日軍戰機後,正在接受急救處理。

Date of Photo 時間:不詳 N/A
Credits 來源:美國國家檔案館 Photo Courtesy of National Archives

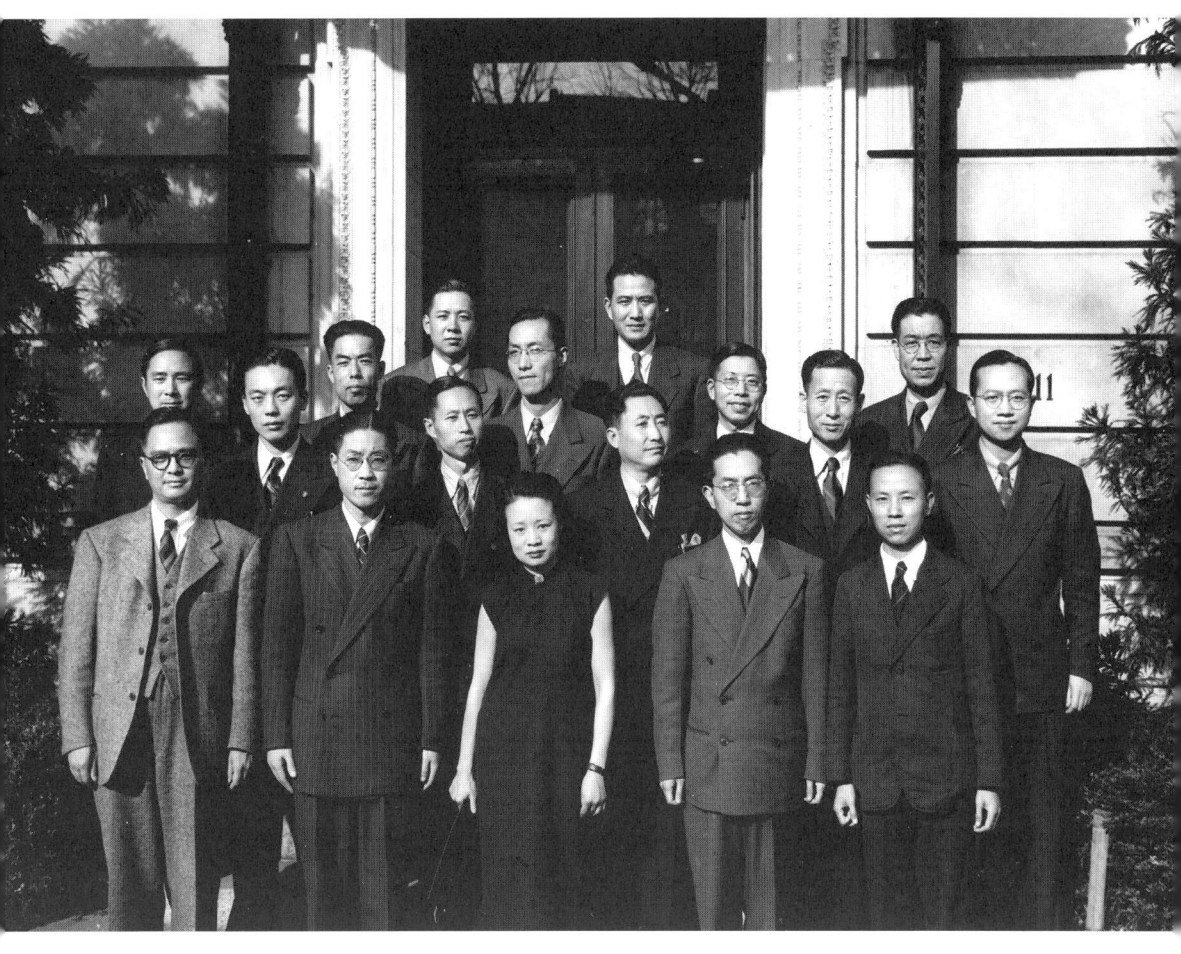

Eighteen Chinese doctors and medical technicians arrived in America, where they stayed for six months to study American medical and health methods under government sponsorship.

十八名中國醫生和專業醫技人員在政府資助下前往美國學習醫療與衛生技術,為期六個月。

Date of Photo 時間:March 21, 1945
Credits 來源:美國國家檔案館 Photo Courtesy of National Archives

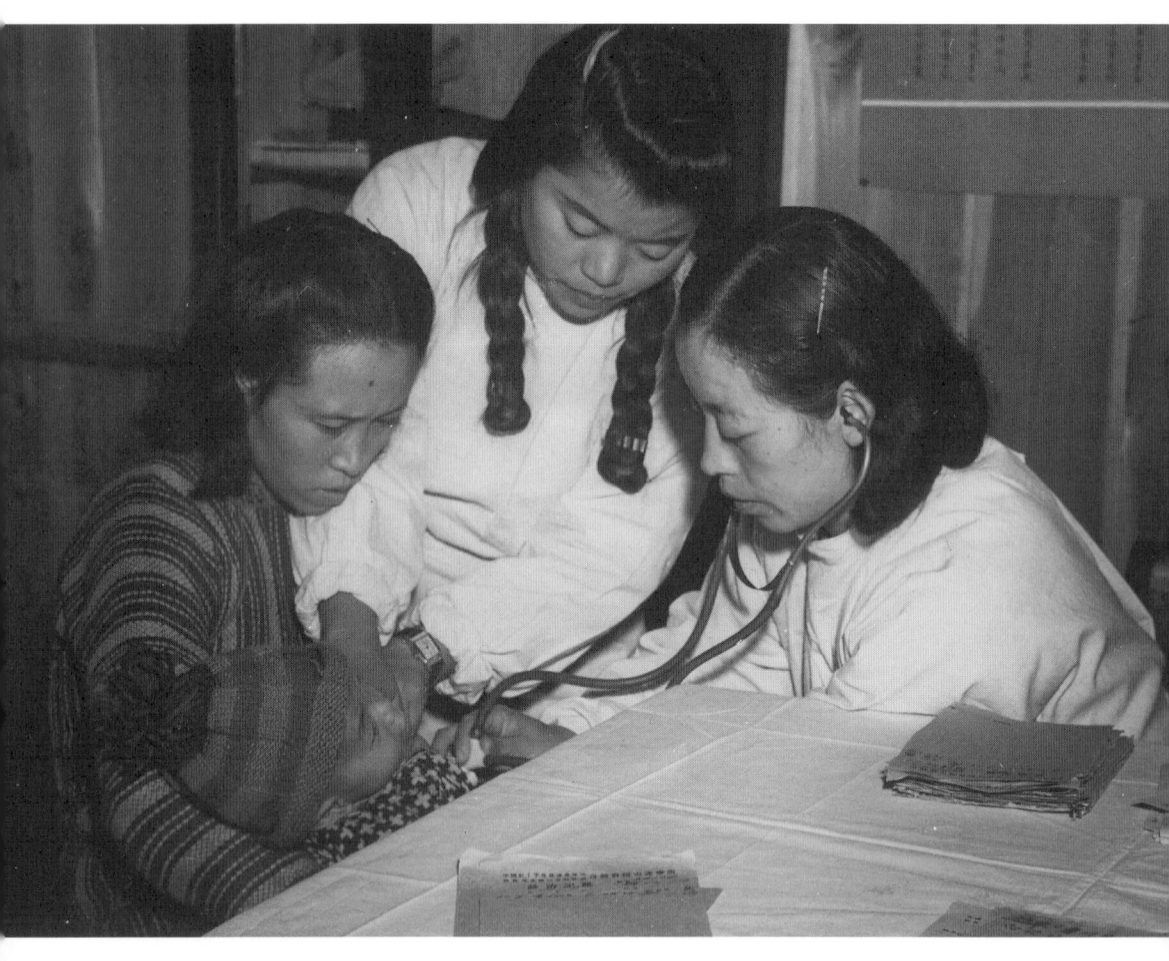

One of China's female doctors checked up on a Chinese baby using the American Red Cross's supplies.

一名中國女醫生使用美國紅十字會提供的物資，為一名中國嬰兒進行檢查。

Date of Photo 時間：不詳 N/A
　　　Credits 來源：美國國家檔案館 Photo Courtesy of National Archives

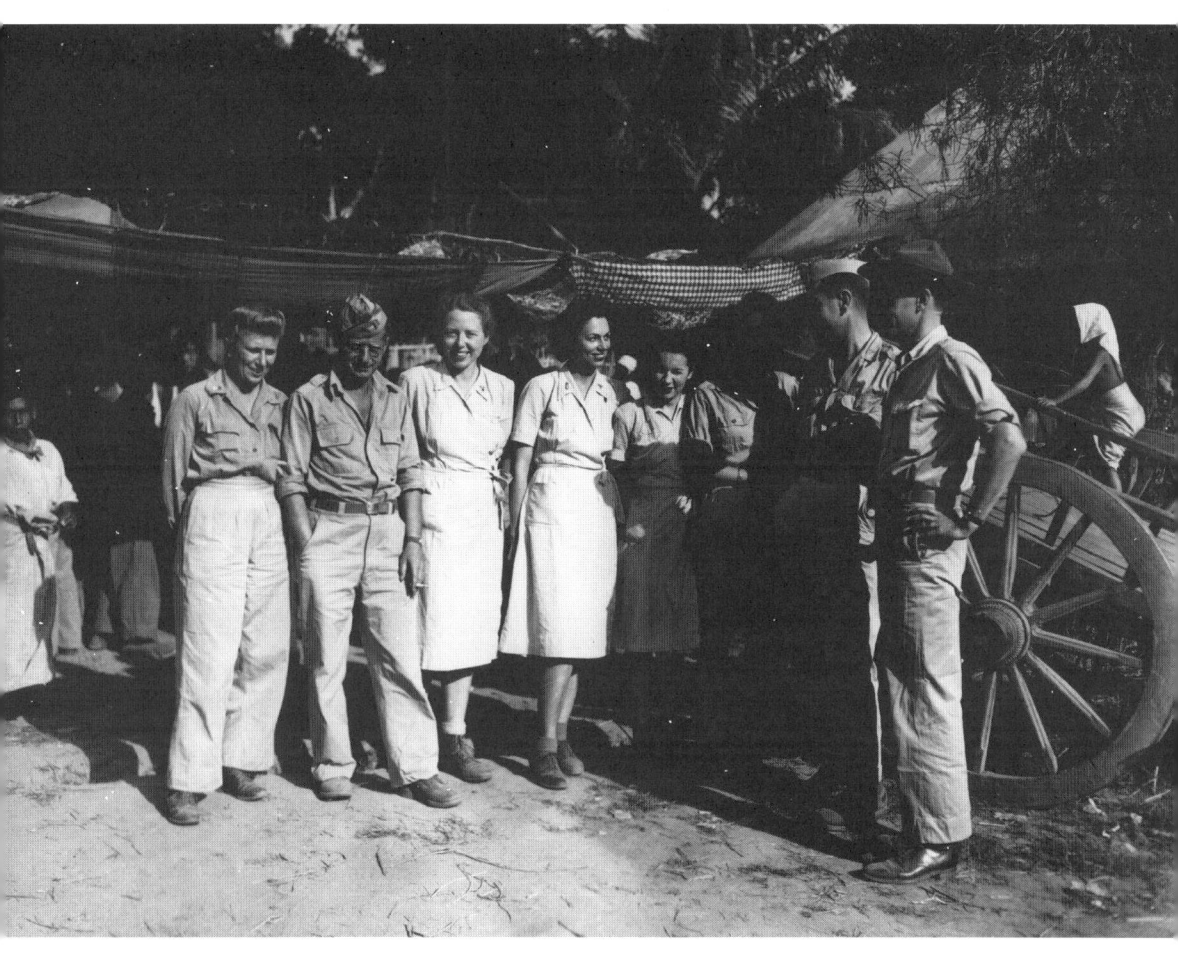

A group photo of nurses and medical officers standing outside the US Army's 44th field hospital at Bhamo, Burma.

一群護理人員與醫療軍官在緬甸八莫的美國陸軍第 44 野戰醫院外合影。

Date of Photo 時間：March 12, 1945
Credits 來源：美國國家檔案館 Photo Courtesy of National Archives

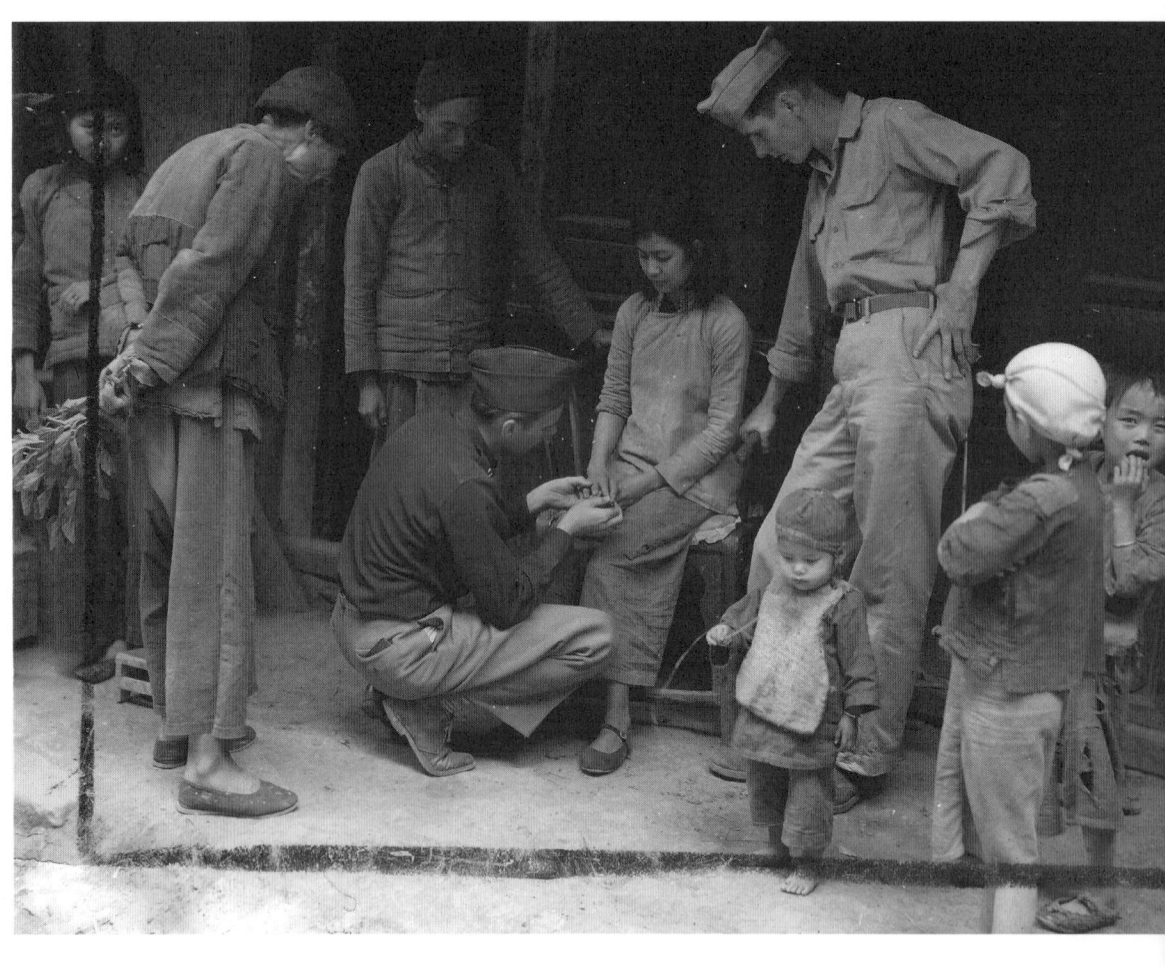

Captain Cullum examines a young Chinese mother, who was suffering from central paralysis.

卡倫上尉為一位癱瘓的年輕中國母親進行檢查。

Date of Photo 時間:不詳 N/A
Credits 來源:美國國家檔案館 Photo Courtesy of National Archives

INFRASTRUCTURE TRANSPORTATION, AND COMMUNICATION

In 1938, the Republic of China boasted a daunting 11.4 million square kilometers of land. And as the Sino-Japanese war picked up and World War II began, China and its foreign helpers, the International Medical Relief Corps (IMRC), came to the harsh realization that the war would not wait for their correspondence. Quick communication and efficient transportation became critical for the continued survival of China against the Japanese. For the International Medical Relief Corps to take decisive action, they needed to make the most of the new, helpful machinery made during the war and also innovate with their existing supplies. They also collaborated extensively with international organizations who provided materials and personnel to the medical forces. The doctors, both Chinese and foreign, struggled together against the ongoing Japanese occupation while fearlessly battling the bureaucracy of their own side, and selflessly devoted their lives to blocking the spread of fascism in China.

Setbacks

One of the many hindrances to the International Medical Relief Corps' cause in China was the ongoing internal conflict between the Chinese Communist Party and the Guomindang Nationalist Party, which often interfered with the communication or intercepted the movement of the IMRC and Dr. Robert Lin, who is the head of the IMRC. In 1939, IMRC doctors Rolf Becker, Bedrich Kisch, and Fritz Jensen contacted Zhou Enlai, the official Chinese Communist Party representative to the Guomindang Nationalist Party, requesting the Guomindang's help in facilitating the transportation of the Chinese Communist Party's Eighth Route Army. Despite the Medical Relief Corps general neutrality, Zhou Enlai denied their request, informing the doctors that the circumstances on the front were not so simple. He instead suggested that these doctors remain on the Guomindang controlled front, with the consolation that no matter where they worked in China, they would be supporting their fight against Japanese aggression.

Indeed, it was near impossible for members of the IMRC to receive permission to assist both the Guomindang and the Chinese Communist Party at the same time. In 1940, doctors David Iancu, Stanislaw Flato, and George Schön went to

Zhou Enlai to voice their concerns, as they felt that they were being forced to work exclusively with the Guomindang Nationalist Party, Dr. David Iancu stated: "It will be almost impossible for me to continue to work with the Guomindang's reactionaries so I asked the Communist Party of Romania for advice. I immediately wrote a letter to Moscow... where I expressed the opinion that it would be preferable to return to my country, then to work with reactionaries. Meanwhile, expecting, along with the others, that our problems would be solved, we returned to the units that we had been assigned to by the Chinese Red Cross." According to Dr. Stanislaw Flato, any access to the Chinese Communist Party in the north was cut off by the Guomindang Nationalist Party, preventing many IMRC members from serving where they truly wished.

Occasionally, the Chinese Communist Party or the Guomindang even sought conflict with the IMRC themselves. In 1940, Dr. Pan Ji of the Guomindang Nationalist Party was appointed as the secretary general of the Chinese Red Cross. But with his leadership, he held the ulterior motive of establishing the Guomindang's political and economic control over the Medical Relief Corps. Dr. Pan Ji employed various tactics to accuse Dr. Lin, of corruption and leftist politics. He took advantage of Dr. Lin's hospitality towards the IMRC's Spanish doctors and his previous cooperation with the Chinese Communist Party to publicly brand him a communist. Following these accusations, Chiang Kai-shek called Dr. Robert Lin to Chongqing, the capital of the wartime nation, in 1940, threatening punishment and demanding that he defend himself from these accusations. Although Dr. Lin escaped this trial relatively unscathed, it would not be the only time that the Medical Relief Corps faced off against the Guomindang Nationalist Party.

After the fall of Hankou, a part of modern-day Wuhan, in 1938, the Chinese armies decided to adopt the strategy of "defending in depth." They aimed to hinder the encroachment of the Imperial Japanese Army by creating a buffer zone —an area completely free of supplies or road infrastructure—so that the Japanese forces would not be able to steal any helpful materials and would be forced to advance their vehicles through land without roads. While they did succeed in slowing the enemy invaders' crawl into central China, it consequently created a medical blockade. The invading army had no path to reach the rest of China, but the IMRC's physicians also had no way to travel to and from the front lines, resulting in a complete lack of medical personnel and supplies for the soldiers now trapped on the front. When the IMRC tried to deliver six tons of medical aid to Yan'an, the Guomindang troops prevented them from entering the city. Despite the IMRC's belief that Chiang Kai-shek had approved of this transport operation, the Guomindang soldiers seized all six tons of their medical supplies, forcing the IMRC to leave Yan'an unsupported and without supplies. This event put a stop to all future attempts to supply the fronts with large quantities of material aid or medicine. After the start of the blockade, Dr. Fritz Jensen even remarked on the constant low capacity of the hospital, stating that the journey from the front line to the field hospital was so perilous that simply arriving at a hospital was an amazing feat. In fact, the reason the IMRC did not place heavy focus on cardiovascular or neurological services was because, most often, none of those patients could survive the perilous trip to the hospital. Journalists of the time estimate that, partially due to the supply blockages, tens of thousands of soldiers and civilians alike perished from lack of proper medication during this war.

More difficulties were encountered within the IMRC continued with Du Yusheng as the vice president of the Chinese Red Cross, whom Swiss journalist Ilona Ralph Sues described as having "a long, egg shaped head, no chin, huge bat like ears, cold cruel lips uncovering big yellow decayed teeth, the sickly complexion of an addict … His eyes were dead and impenetrable …He gave me his limp cold hand. A huge bony hand with two inch long, brown opium-stained claws." Despite Du Yusheng's support of the Chinese Red Cross' scientists and doctors, his true allegiances remained with the Green Gang, a Shanghainese criminal organization and secret society which influenced social and political movements in China throughout the 20th century. He used his influential position to place unreasonable restrictions on Dr. Robert Lin and the IMRC, presenting yet another challenge to the Corps' operations during this time.

If the political pressure from the Chinese Communist Party and the Guomindang were not enough, the IMRC also faced countless physical obstacles with China's rigorous terrain. When the need arose for The Chinese Red Cross to provide aid in Shaanxi, many units expressed reluctance on taking up the mission simply because the path took them across the treacherous Yellow River. Yu Tao-Chen, a member of the 61st unit of the Chinese Red Cross and IMRC explained that, "Everyone has a burning desire to cross the Yellow River, but once crossed; then tears will flow, for one realizes the dangers which have to be surmounted on returning." Certainly, the harrowing journey across the river kept many units from the front lines. But if the unforgiving waters of the Yellow River were not enough to dissuade the Medical Relief Corps members, the perilous journey and ever-present risk of dying to the Imperial Japanese Army firmly dampened the doctors' hopes for the journey. While outright oppression from political forces hindered the IMRC's movement, the general peril of travelling through a warzone made on unfamiliar land factored into the transportation troubles of the Corps.

Communication

The medical fields of the United States and China had a cooperative friendship. Upon Dr. Robert Lin's arrival to the United States, he consulted the Surgeon General of the United States Army, Norman T. Kirk, to gather new ideas for the medical service, which he promptly brought back to the Chinese Army. For his service in supporting China, and therefore the allied powers, in the war, President Franklin D. Roosevelt awarded him with the Legion of Merit in 1944.

The United States and China also collaborated on programs such as the United States Army Chinese Combat Command led by General A. C. Wedemeyer, the commander of American forces in the Chinese Theater. The goal of this initiative was for the American forces to provide professional training and tactical advice for the Chinese armies, as well as to equip them with adequate combat equipment. Notably, they also facilitated medical education to the Chinese, allowing for the training of more field doctors and nurses who would become vital towards the war effort.

The most prominent challenges with Sino-American communications were, predictably, the language barrier and the physical distance between the two lands. Designated translators and bilingual army members were able to partially bridge the gap between English and Chinese communication. One such person happened to be Dr. Robert Lin. Being born of Chinese parentage while growing up in Scotland lent Dr. Robot Lin a unique linguistic background which helped him to properly facilitate the Corps according to the needs of both the Chinese and American troops. The physical distance was bridged with the relatively new development of reliable radio technology. Individual platoons had radio equipment which allowed for seamless short-distance communication. But fulfilling the army's need for overseas communications gave way to the development of the Radio Teletype, a device which used radio connections to display typed messages between two or more terminals. Inspired by the pre-existing landline teleprinter operations, these machines were composed of three main components: the teleprinter, the modem, and the radio. The teleprinter contained a keyboard and a printer by which one could type out and view messages. The modem is an electronic device located between the teleprinter and the radio transceiver, which translates the digital signal from the teleprinter to audio frequency signals when sending out a message. Even though the Radio Teletype was many years in the making, its development significantly bolstered the Chinese war efforts by facilitating efficient communication between the Chinese forces and their American collaborators.

Transportation

The war never stopped moving and, as a result, the IMRC's physicians had to adapt to a lighter lifestyle to accommodate for their constant travel. One such adaptation was the bedrolls, or pugai, which was comparable to a modern-day sleeping bag. These bedrolls managed to condense an entire sleeping set-up including a mat, pillows, bedsheets, and mosquito nets into a single compact package which was hung and carried on bamboo rods. Even when the group lacked pack animals to carry cargo, local civilians were often very willing to assist the medics in small-scale transportation projects. These locals' intimate knowledge of the local terrain allowed them to assist doctors in boating across rivers, whacking through forests, and general navigation. The peasants assigned to support the unit shocked the IMRC's physicians by easily lifting up to 45 kilograms of cargo almost 30 kilometers a day.

The C-47 aircraft, developed in 1941, was key to the success of the Allied forces in the China-Burma-India Theater. They were constructed in the American west coast, and American troops brought these crafts to China in their contribution to the war effort. Compared to the C-53 aircraft, the C-47 was outfitted with a fitted cargo door, hoist attachments, and glider-towing capabilities. Although the vessel's size was not dramatically larger than its predecessors, the fitted door let it carry a much wider range of cargo than previously possible, simply due to the fact that it could fit larger items through the doors. Additionally, the ability to tow gliders proved vital in rescue operations. Although it had no value as a combat craft, these traits made it the most reliable plane for transporting cargo, troops, and the wounded during the war. Because of its outstanding mobility and compact form, the C-47 was indispensable in moving against the ambulant Japanese Army and in navigating the dense jungles of New Guinea and Burma. As seen through the large-scale removal of wounded soldiers from the Myitkyina Front, the Chinese forces used the C-47 crafts extensively in rescue missions and for transporting wounded soldiers from the front lines to various field hospitals for further treatment.

When the road infrastructure was kind, the IMRC could use the American Dodge WC-54 ambulances to move injured personnel. Weighing almost a ton, these vehicles could accommodate a driver, a medic, and four to seven other passengers. The interior of the vehicle held four fold-away bunks which could transport patients lying down but could also be folded away to fit more non-critical patients. For the comfort of the passengers, these ambulances also had heaters embedded into their fireproof walls and a foldaway step to the rear entrance. Although they did not have the amenities of a modern ambulance, the WC-54s often had buckets or containers of emergency medical supplies and a spare wheel attached to the side.

Although most of these vehicles were supplied by the United States Military, it was frequent practice for Americans to express support for the Chinese front by raising money and sponsoring military crafts, many of which were designed and manufactured in the United States. An example of this occurred in 1945, when the students of Barber School in Detroit, Michigan donated an L-5 liaison plane nicknamed the "Angel of Mercy" to the troops in China, which would later be piloted by Sergeant Arthur H. Van Wye and rescue soldiers from the front lines in Synthe, Burma.

Where these vehicles could not reach, however, the Chinese forces compensated by using the native oxen for transport. Oxen have been domesticated in China for over 2,000 years, so the Medical Corps took advantage of their natural ability to maneuver through the land and their impressive pulling capacity of almost 1,700 pounds to transport cargo and injured soldiers. Countless soldiers were saved on the back of these oxen, as seen through the successful evacuation of the Chinese soldiers after a skirmish with the Japanese at Myitkyina. The oxen, led by the medical forces and the non-injured troops, carried the wounded over five miles of worn, muddy road from the battle's front lines to the Myitkyina air strip, where they were quickly loaded onto the waiting C-47 aircrafts and transferred to the safety of the nearby 18th field hospitals on Ledo Road, Myitkyina.

The expeditionary forces in China also used mules as pack animals, due to their ability to carry up to ninety kilograms of dead weight, and 160 kilograms of live weight. Previously prominent in China's commerce industry, the mule was now being used to transport medical aid from base to base. As Major Charles B. Randall of the Timberland, North Carolina Veterinary Corps suggested to General R. A. Kellser, the troops in Ramgarh, India could make use of the available mule population to create a pack train and transport their medical supplies. At the Ramgarh Training Center, soldiers of the 669th Quartermaster Remount Troop even kept organized file record cards on the branding numbers, physical descriptions, breeding histories, and medical records of each individual mule.

Infrastructure

Unsurprisingly, China's wartime hospital infrastructure varied greatly from hospital to hospital. In the Shaanxi province, for example, the IMRC inhabited the Canadian-American International Peace Hospital, which was carved into the face of a local mountain. From the exterior, the hospital seemed to be a series of holes carved out of the mountain range, shielded with wrought metallic doorways. The trellis design which the engineers dug into the side of the mountain created multiple stories or levels in this hospital, allowing a single section of the mountain to accommodate nearly 30 rooms. On the inside, the hospital was quite successful, caring for thousands of wounded Chinese throughout the war. Although the location may initially seem dubious, the natural geography proved extremely useful, the mountain's innate stability protecting the hospital through and withstanding multiple Japanese bombings.

In Burma, the IMRC physicians found work in an evacuation hospital nicknamed the "Bamboo Bowl Theater" because it was made completely with thin, woven bamboo sheets. This building's exterior walls, standing over twenty feet in height, were constructed entirely with the woven bamboo sheets which protected the treatment facilities from the outside dust. The pointed hip-style roof, covered fully with large tarps, gave the hospital protection from the sun and rain, and provided natural cooling by encouraging air flow. Because the IMRC worked mostly in pre-existing hospitals, the hospital infrastructures which were available to them included buildings of varying size, quality, and equipment. Still, at whichever hospital the volunteer physicians were stationed at, they worked to the best of their ability to fulfill the medical needs of the soldiers and civilians of the resistance.

基礎建設、
運輸、通訊

1938年，中華民國傲然擁有一片廣袤無垠的土地，疆域達一千一百四十萬平方公里。隨著中日戰爭持續升溫及第二次世界大戰的爆發，中國與其外國援助者（亦即國際醫療救護隊）意識到殘酷的現實處境：戰爭不會因為他們需要時間關係而停下腳步。因此，快速的通訊與高效的運輸成為了中國持續對抗日軍的關鍵。而為了能夠果斷採取行動，國際醫療救護隊必須充分運用戰時製造出的新型設備，並在現有物資的基礎上進行創新。他們也與眾多國際組織密切合作，從中獲得物資與人員支援，投入醫療工作。這些中外醫生一同在日軍持續佔領的壓力下奮戰，面對敵軍時無所畏懼，且勇敢與本方體制內的官僚體制鬥爭，他們無私地將生命致力於阻止法西斯主義在中國的蔓延。

困境與阻礙

　　國際醫療救護隊在中國面臨的眾多障礙之一，便是中共與國民黨之間持續的內部衝突，這時常妨礙醫療救護隊的溝通，或阻礙國際醫療救護隊及其負責人林可勝博士的行動。1939年，國際醫療救護隊的醫生白樂夫（Rolf Becker）、紀瑞德（Bedrich Kisch）和嚴斐德（Fritz Jensen）聯絡周恩來，因為他是中共派駐國民黨統治地區的代表，希望他能請求國民黨協助包括他在內的許多外籍醫生前往中共八路軍所在的前線地區。儘管國際醫療救護隊保持中立，周恩來仍拒絕了他們的請求，並告訴這些醫生，前線的情況並不簡單。他冷淡地建議這些醫生留在國民黨控制的前線，並安慰他們，無論他們在哪裡工作，都是在支援中國對抗日本的侵略。

　　確實，國際醫療救護隊的成員幾乎不可能獲准同時幫助國民黨與中共。1940年，外籍醫生楊固（David Iancu）、柯理格（Stanislaw Flato）和沈恩拜訪周恩來表達他們的擔憂，因為他們感覺自己被迫僅與國民黨合作。楊固醫生表示：「對我來說，繼續與國民黨政府合作幾乎是不可能的，因此我向羅馬尼亞共產黨尋求建議。我立即寫信至莫斯科，我在信中提及，與其和國民黨政府合作我不如歸返祖國。與此同時，我和其他人一樣，期待著我們的問題能夠得到解決，於是我們返回了中國紅十字會分配給我們的單位。」根據醫生楊固的說法，國民黨全面切斷了前往北方共產黨控制區的道路，使許多國際醫療救護隊成員無法在他們真正希望服務的地區行醫。

有時，中共或國民黨甚至會直接和國際醫療救護隊發生衝突。1940年，國民黨的潘驥博士（即潘小萼）獲任命為中國紅十字會秘書長，但他的領導背後懷有別有用心的動機——他企圖將國民黨的政經控制力量擴張至國際醫療救護隊。潘驥博士用盡手段，指控國際醫療救護隊負責人林可勝博士貪腐並支持左翼政治。他利用林可勝博士對西班牙醫生的熱情接待，以及他過去與中共的合作，公開將他扣上「親共」的帽子。遭受此一指控之後，蔣中正於 1940 年將林可勝博士召往陪都重慶，威脅要懲處他，並要求他為自己辯護。儘管林可勝博士最終安然逃過一劫，但這只是國民黨刻意為難國際醫療救護隊的種種作為之一。

1938 年，隨著漢口（今武漢的一部分）淪陷，中國軍隊決定採取「縱深防禦」的戰略。他們試圖建立一個緩衝區（亦即完全沒有物資或道路基礎設施的區域），藉此阻止日軍的推進，使其無法劫掠任何補給物，並被迫在沒有道路的地形上艱難行進。這一策略確實成功延緩了日軍向中國腹地的推進，但同時也造成了醫療封鎖。侵略的日軍無法進一步深入中國，而國際醫療救護隊的醫生也無法往返前線，導致前線士兵陷入了無醫無藥的絕境。國際醫療救護隊試圖運送六噸醫療物資至延安，遭國民黨軍隊阻止，無法進入。儘管蔣中正已批准此次運輸行動，但國民黨的軍隊仍然將這批醫療物資沒收，救護隊只能無奈離開，延安前線因此陷入了孤立無援的境地。此次事件過後，再也沒有人嘗試向前線運送大規模醫療物資。實行封鎖後，外籍醫生嚴斐德甚至感嘆他的野戰醫院始終沒有很多病人可以收治，因為從前線抵達該醫院的路程極為險峻，能夠活著到達醫院就已經很了不起了。其實，國際醫療救護隊之所以沒有將重點放在心血管或神經科醫療上，正是因為大多數這類病患根本無法活著撐過這段危險的路程。當時的新聞記者估計，受這些供應封鎖影響，因缺乏適當醫療而在戰爭中喪生的士兵和平民可說是數以萬計。

國際醫療救護隊在運作的過程中還面臨著來自內部的挑戰，尤其是在杜月笙擔任中國紅十字會副會長期間。瑞士記者伊洛娜・拉爾夫・蘇斯（Ilona Ralph Sues）曾這樣描述杜月笙：「他的頭是狹長的蛋形，沒有下巴，長著一對巨大的蝙蝠耳，冷酷的嘴唇掩不住一口黃色爛牙，膚色像是個病人，宛如一名癮君子⋯⋯他的雙眼死寂而深不可測⋯⋯他向我伸出他那隻冰冷無力的手，一隻枯瘦如柴的大手，指甲長達兩英寸，泛著棕色的鴉片污漬。」儘管杜月笙曾支持中國紅十字會的科學家和醫生，但他的真正效忠對象卻始終是青幫——整個20世紀影響著中國社會與政治運動的上海幫會。他利用自己在紅十字會的影響力對林可勝博士及國際醫療救護隊施加種種不合理的限制，使救護隊的運作更加困難。

然而，國際醫療救護隊面臨的不僅是來自中共與國民黨的政治壓力，還有中國險峻地形帶來的無數困難。當中國紅十字會要向陝西提供援助時，許多醫療團隊對此任務望而卻步，唯一的理由就是他們不想穿越險惡的黃河。中國紅十字會第61醫療隊及國際醫療救護隊成員余道真[1]曾如此形容這一旅程：「每個人都懷抱著對黃河彼岸的熱烈渴望，一旦渡過卻又會落淚，因為這時才真正意識到歸途中將要克服重重險阻。」無庸置疑的，這趟跋山涉水且險阻重重的路程使許多醫療隊無法抵達前線。然而，若黃河洶湧的水勢尚不足以令醫療救護隊的成員卻步，那麼戰場上的危機四伏與日軍的殘暴威脅，則讓這段旅程變得愈加令人絕望。在政治因素壓迫使國際醫療救護隊舉步維艱的同時，戰爭的殘酷現實與對異國土地的陌生感，也讓這支醫療隊在交通運輸的安排上遇到許多困難。

戰時通訊

中美醫界一直保持著合作與友誼。林可勝博士抵達美國後，特意拜訪了美國陸軍軍醫署署長諾曼・柯克（Norman T. Kirk），以汲取新的醫療服務理念，並迅速將這些創新思維帶回中國軍隊。由於他對中國的對日抗戰有卓越功勳，等於間接援助同盟國，美國總統羅斯福於1944年授予他功績勳章。

---

[1] 是北京協和醫學院畢業的中國護理先驅。

此外，中美兩國還在多個項目上展開合作，其中包括由美國駐中國戰區司令官，即陸軍將領魏德邁（A. C. Wedemeyer）指揮的美軍中國戰區作戰司令部（United States Army Chinese Combat Command）。該計畫的目標是由美軍為中國軍隊提供專業訓練與戰術指導，同時協助配發充足的戰鬥裝備。值得注意的是，該計畫還促進了中國的醫學教育，使更多戰地醫生與護士得以接受培訓，成為戰爭期間至關重要的醫療支援力量。

中美交流面臨的最大挑戰，不外乎主要是語言障礙和兩國之間的遙遠距離。為了彌合這一鴻溝，特派的翻譯人員與精通雙語的軍隊成員在一定程度上促進了英語和漢語之間的溝通。其中一位關鍵人物便是林可勝博士。由於他出生於華人家庭，卻在蘇格蘭長大，這使他具備獨特的語言背景，能夠根據中美雙方軍隊的需求協調國際醫療救護隊的運作。

而隨著無線電技術的發展，也逐步克服了物理距離。每個分隊都配有無線電設備，使短距離通訊得以流暢進行。然而，要滿足軍隊對跨國溝通的需求，則促使「無線電電傳打字機」（Radio Teletype）的發展。這種設備利用無線電波連接多個終端裝置，顯示鍵盤輸入的訊息，靈感來源於早期的有線電傳打字機系統。無線電電傳打字機主要由三個部分組成：電傳機、數據機和無線電收發機。電傳機配有鍵盤與印表機，負責輸出與顯示訊息。數據機則位於電傳機與無線電收發機之間，負責將電傳機的數字信號轉換為可傳輸的音頻信號，從而發送訊息。儘管這項技術經過多年研發才得以真正使用，但它的誕生極大地增強了中國的戰時通訊能力，提升中國軍隊與美軍協同作戰的效率。

戰地運輸

無休止的戰爭迫使國際醫療救護隊的醫生們適應了輕便的生活模式，以應對不斷遷徙的需求。其中一項重要的適應措施便是「舖蓋」，其功能類似於現代的睡袋。這些舖蓋將整套睡眠設備，包括墊子、枕頭、床單與蚊帳都壓縮成一個小巧的包裹，並可掛在竹竿上攜帶，即便沒有馱獸，自己也能輕鬆隨身攜帶。此外，當地百姓經常自願協助醫療隊運輸物資，為醫生們提供寶貴的支援。這些百姓憑藉對地形的熟悉，幫助醫療隊划船渡河、開闢叢林道路，並提供簡單的導航指引。更令國際醫療救護隊醫生們震驚的是，這些農民能夠輕鬆揹負多達 45 公斤的貨物並日行近 30 公里，展現出驚人的體能與韌性。

C-47 運輸機於 1941 年研製，成為中緬印戰區（CBI 戰區）盟軍成功的關鍵之一。這些飛機在美國西岸製造，隨後由美軍運往中國，為戰爭貢獻力量。與 C-53 運輸機相比，C-47 配備了加固貨艙門、起重設備，以及拖曳滑翔機使用的設備。儘管其機身尺寸與前代機型差異不大，但由於貨艙門更寬，使其能載運比以往更大型的物資。此外，其滑翔機拖曳能力在救援行動中發揮了至關重要的作用。雖然 C-47 並非戰鬥機，但憑藉卓越的機動性和適應性，成為戰時最可靠的運輸機，負責運送補給、部隊及傷患。尤其在緬甸與新幾內亞的叢林作戰中，C-47 的靈活性使其能夠有效應對活動能力強大的日軍。例如，C-47 能從密支那前線將大量傷兵撤離至後方野戰醫院接受治療。

道路條件良好時，國際醫療救護隊則會使用美製道奇 WC-54 救護車運送傷員。這款救護車重約一噸，可搭載一名駕駛員、一名醫護人員，並容納四至七名傷患。車內設有四張可折疊病床，可供傷患平躺，若將病床折起，則能容納更多輕傷病患。為了提高乘坐舒適度，WC-54 還配備了內嵌式暖氣、防火牆板，以及可折疊的後門踏板。雖然其設備無法與現代救護車相比，但車上通常會攜帶緊急醫療補給桶，並在車身側面裝有備用輪胎，以備不時之需。

儘管大多數軍用車輛由美國軍方供應，但美國民間也經常透過籌款和贊助方式，捐贈許多由美國設計和製造的軍用設備，以支持中國前線的軍事行動。例如，密西根州底特律的巴伯學校（Barber School）[2] 學生於 1945 年募資捐贈了一架 L-5 聯絡機，並將其命名為「仁慈天使號」（Angel of Mercy）。這架飛機後來由美軍飛行員亞瑟・范懷（Sergeant Arthur H. Van Wye）駕駛，在緬甸新題（Synthe）前線成功營救受傷士兵。

---

2 不確定是否為理髮學校，因此用音譯。

然而，當這些車輛無法抵達某些偏遠地區時，中國軍隊則依靠當地的耕牛來滿足運輸需求。中國馴養農耕用牛隻已有兩千多年歷史，因此醫療部隊充分利用耕牛對當地地形的適應性，以及其強大的負重能力來運送傷患。（可拉動近 1700 磅的貨物或人員。）無數士兵因此得以獲救，例如在密支那與日軍交戰後，醫療隊與未受傷的部隊成員利用耕牛將傷患運送超過五英里，穿越泥濘崎嶇的道路，抵達密支那機場。隨後，傷患被迅速安置在待命中的 C-47 運輸機上，並轉送至緬甸利多公路（Ledo Road，即中印公路）附近的第 18 野戰醫院，接受緊急救治。

除了耕牛，中國遠征軍還廣泛徵用騾子當作運輸工具，因為這種馱獸能夠負載的靜負載（dead weight）高達 90 公斤，活負載（live weight）甚至可達到 160 公斤。[3] 過去在中國商業運輸中發揮重要作用的騾子，戰時則被改用於運送醫療物資。來自北卡羅萊納州廷伯蘭獸醫兵團（Veterinary Corps）的獸醫軍官查爾斯·蘭德爾少校（Major Charles B. Randall）向 R.A. 凱爾瑟將軍（R. A. Kellser）提出建議後，駐紮於印度藍姆伽（Ramgarh）的部隊開始籌組專用於醫療補給運輸的騾隊。在藍姆伽訓練中心，669 軍需補給隊（669th Quartermaster Remount Troop）甚至為每頭騾子建立了詳細的檔案，記錄騾子身上烙印的編號、外貌特徵、血統歷史及醫療紀錄，確保這些寶貴的運輸資源能夠得到妥善管理與調配。

基礎建設

中國各地的戰時醫院基礎設施條件理所當然參差不齊。在陝西省，國際醫療救護隊駐紮於加美國際和平醫院（Canadian-American International Peace Hospital），這座醫院並非傳統建築，而是巧妙地嵌入當地山體之中。從外部來看，醫院如同隱匿於山壁的洞窟群，每個入口以鍛造金屬門加固，低調而堅固。工程師們採用棚架式設計，在山體側面開鑿出多層結構，使這片岩壁能夠容納近 30 個病房，形成了獨特的

---

3 死重是指純粹貨物的重量，因為密度比較扎實，背起來比較重。活重則是指活物的重量，例如人的重量。

醫療空間。儘管醫院外觀簡陋,其內部運作效率卻相當高,戰時救治了千千萬萬中國傷患。這樣的選址初看或許顯得奇怪,但其地理條件反而提供了關鍵優勢。堅硬的山體不僅確保了建築的穩定性,還有效抵禦了日軍的歷次空襲威脅。

在緬甸,國際醫療救護隊的醫師們在一座後方醫院中工作,該醫院因為以單薄而綿密的竹片建造而獲得「竹碗手術室」(Bamboo Bowl Theater)的別稱。這座建築的外牆高達二十英尺,全以編織竹片構成,能有效防止室外塵土進入醫療設施。其尖頂式的屋頂被大型防水布完全覆蓋著,不僅能遮陽避雨,更透過設計引導氣流,達到自然降溫的效果。由於國際醫療救護隊大多在既有的醫院中工作,這些可利用的醫療基礎設施在規模、品質及設備上參差不齊。然而,無論這些醫師們獲派前往哪裡當志工,他們都竭盡所能,滿足抗戰士兵與平民的醫療需求。

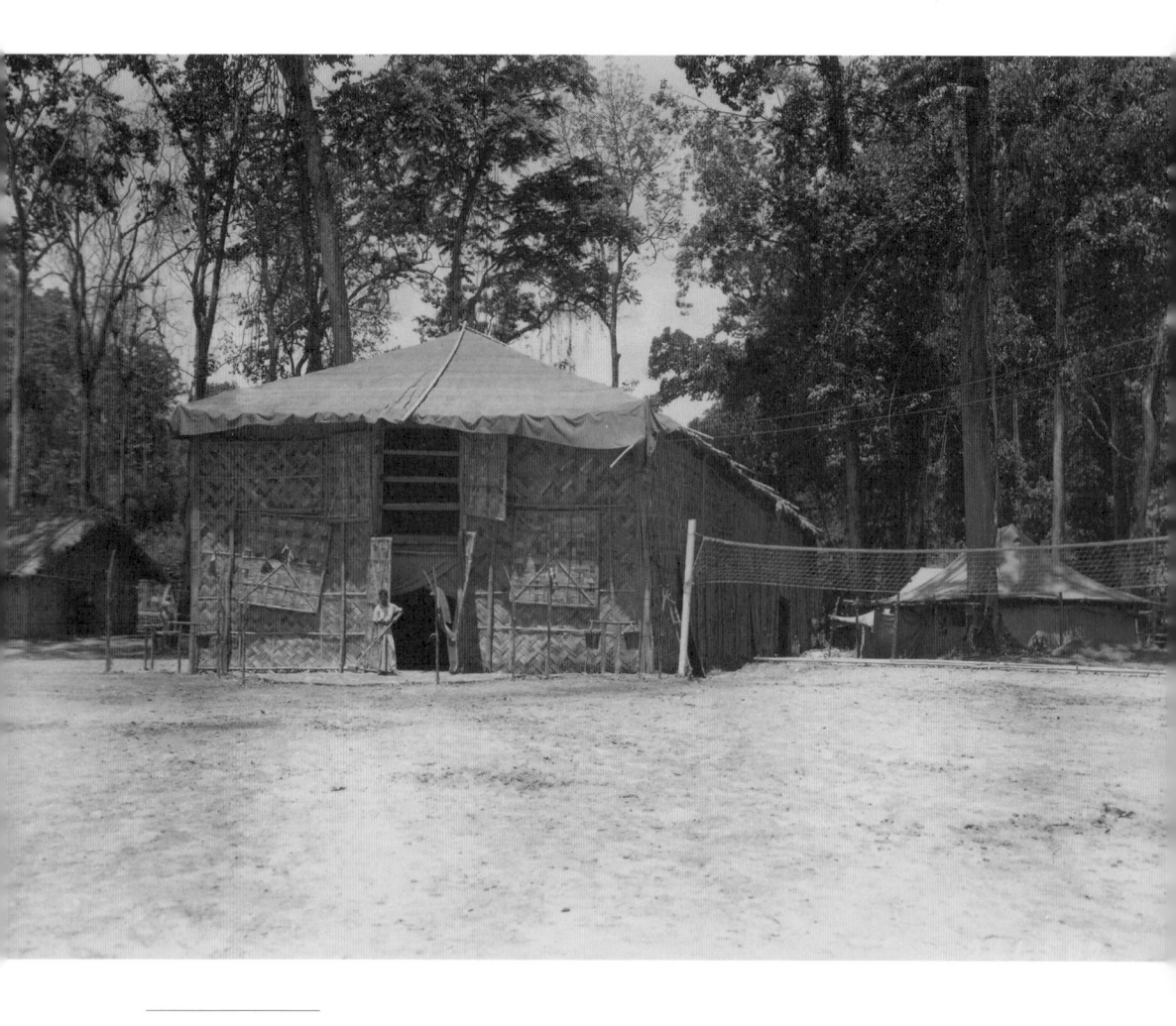

An operating theater nicknamed The Bamboo Bowl located at one of the US Army Evacuation Hospitals in Burma.

位於緬甸某美國陸軍後送醫院院區的手術室,有「竹碗」的別號。

Date of Photo 時間:May 21, 1944
Credits 來源:美國國家檔案館 Photo Courtesy of National Archives

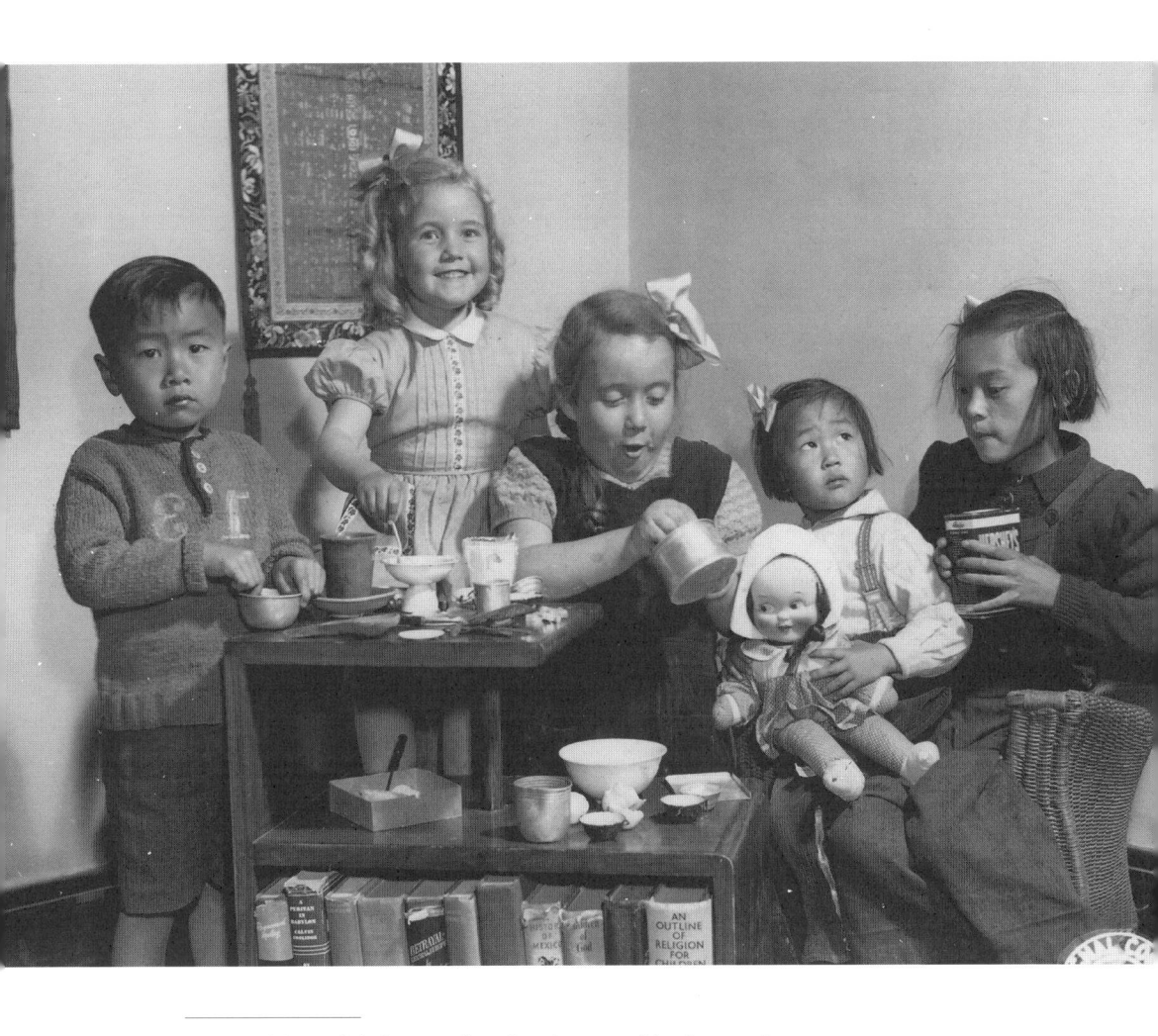

Four children of different cultural and national backgrounds having fun at a tea party.

四名來自不同文化和國家的兒童在茶會上歡樂相聚。

Date of Photo 時間:January 30, 1945
Credits 來源:美國國家檔案館 Photo Courtesy of National Archives

Dr. Donald D. Van Slyke greeted Dr. Robert Lin upon his arrival to the United States.

唐諾‧范斯萊克博士在林可勝博士抵達美國時親自與他見面。

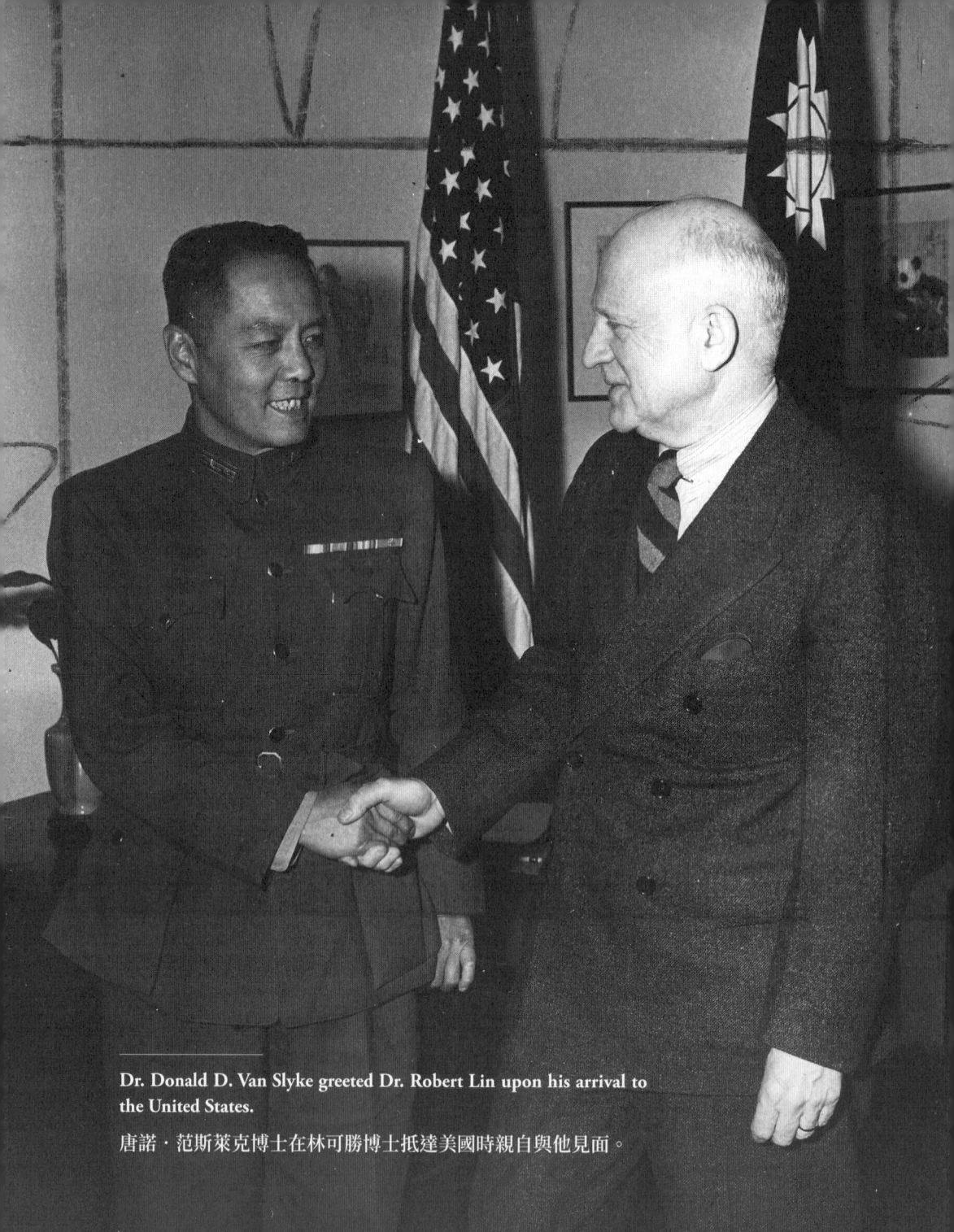

Date of Photo 時間：April 7, 1944
Credits 來源：美國國家檔案館 Photo Courtesy of National Archives

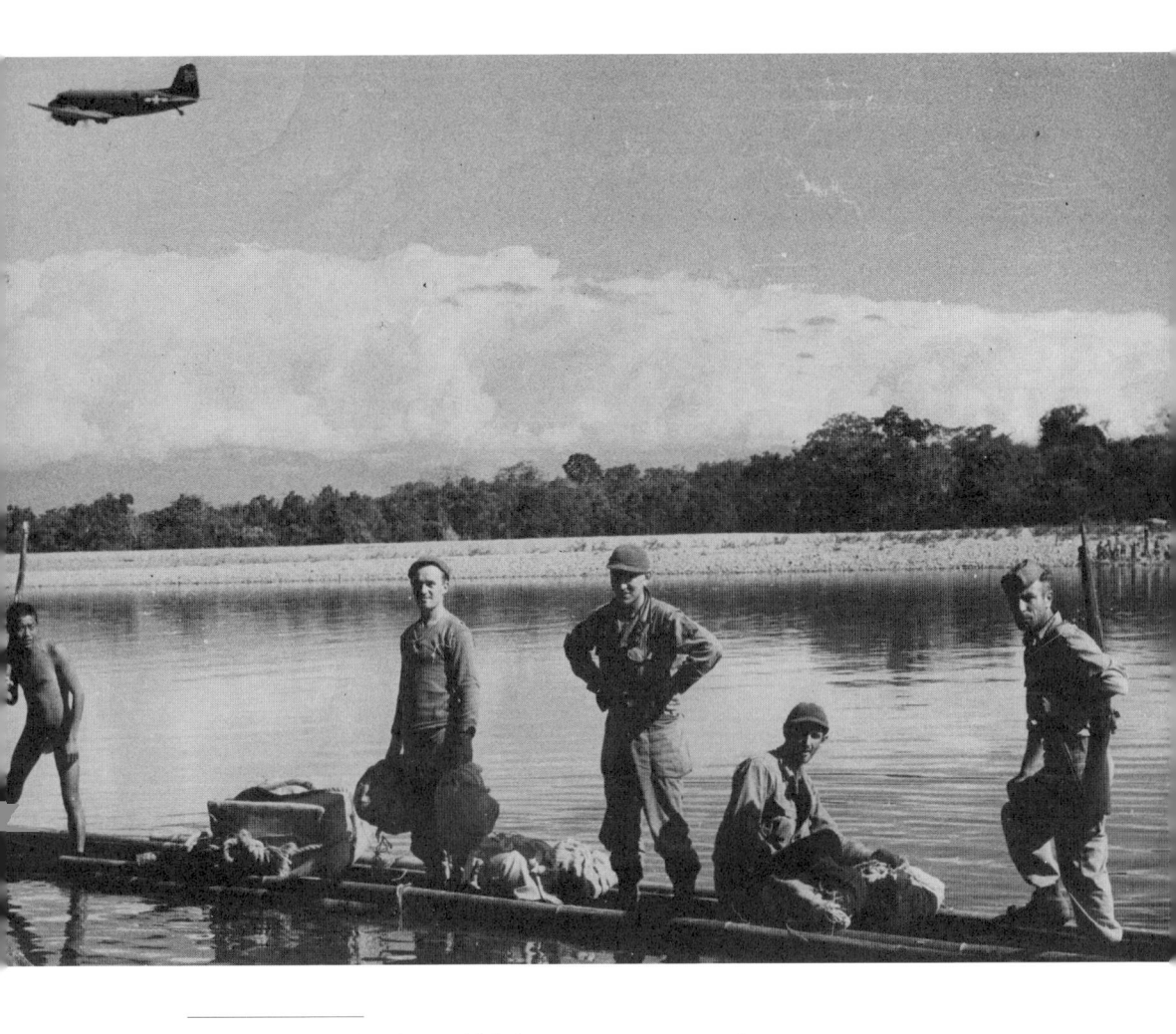

Several Chinese locals would help American privates boat across a river.

數名中國當地居民協助美國士兵划船渡河。

Date of Photo 時間：January 20, 1944
Credits 來源：美國國家檔案館 Photo Courtesy of National Archives

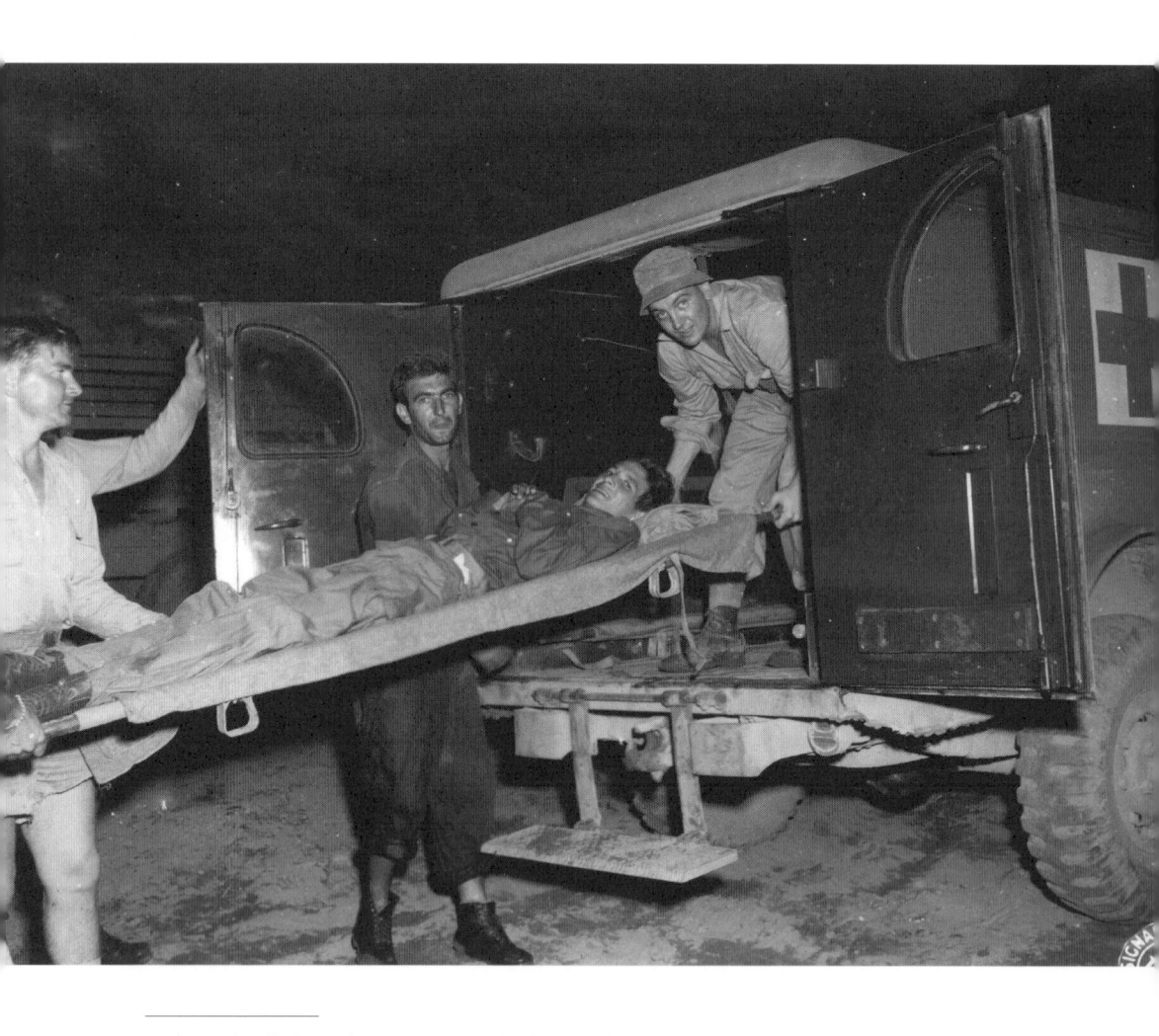

Helpers loaded a pilot into an ambulance after a rescue mission.

救援行動結束後,救援人員將一名飛行員抬上救護車。

Date of Photo 時間:September 13, 1944
Credits 來源:美國國家檔案館 Photo Courtesy of National Archives

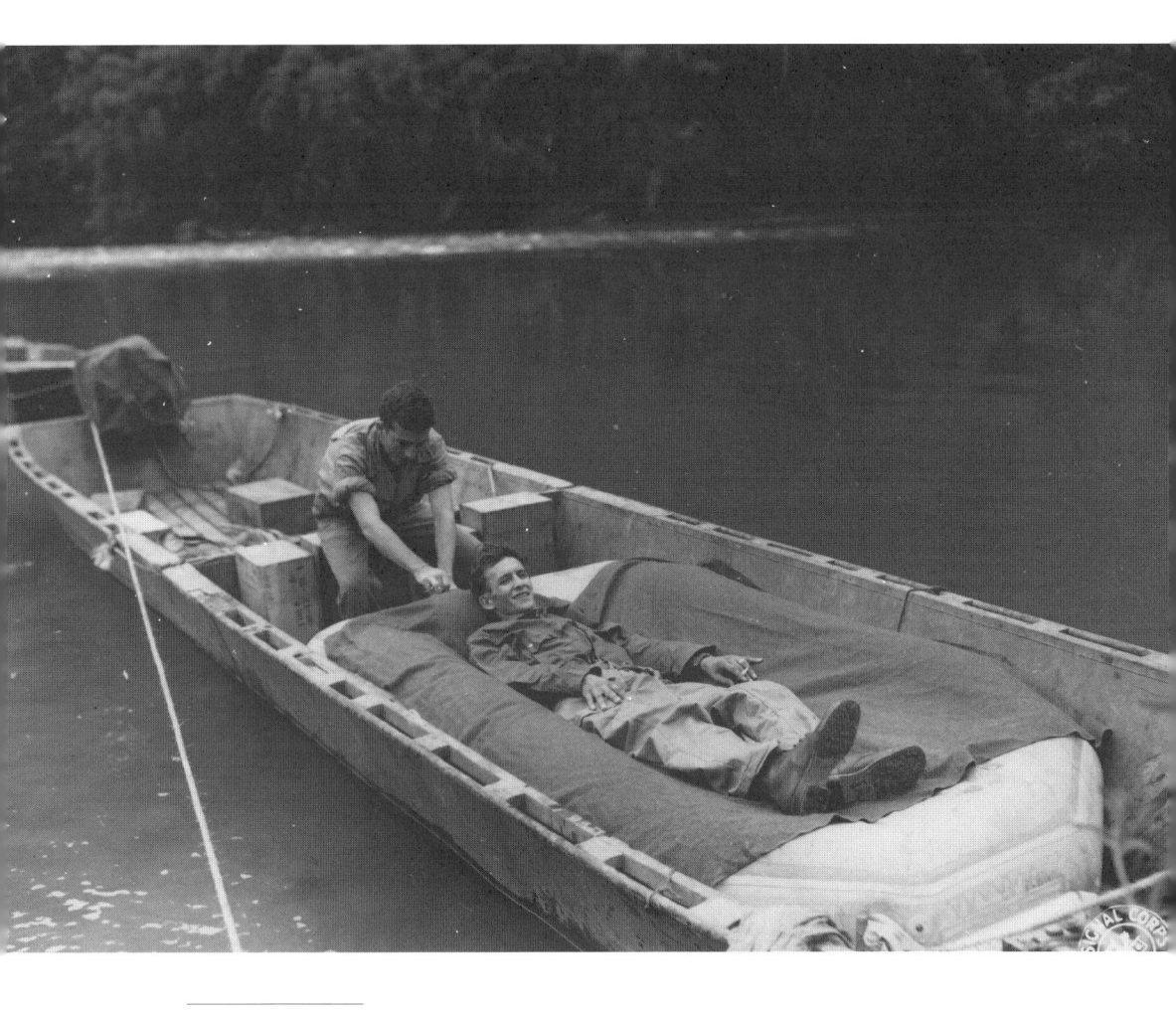

An injured Lieutenant was floated out of a jungle on his way to the hospital.

一名受傷的中尉被抬上小船,將穿越叢林被送往醫院。

Date of Photo 時間：September 13, 1944
Credits 來源：美國國家檔案館 Photo Courtesy of National Archives

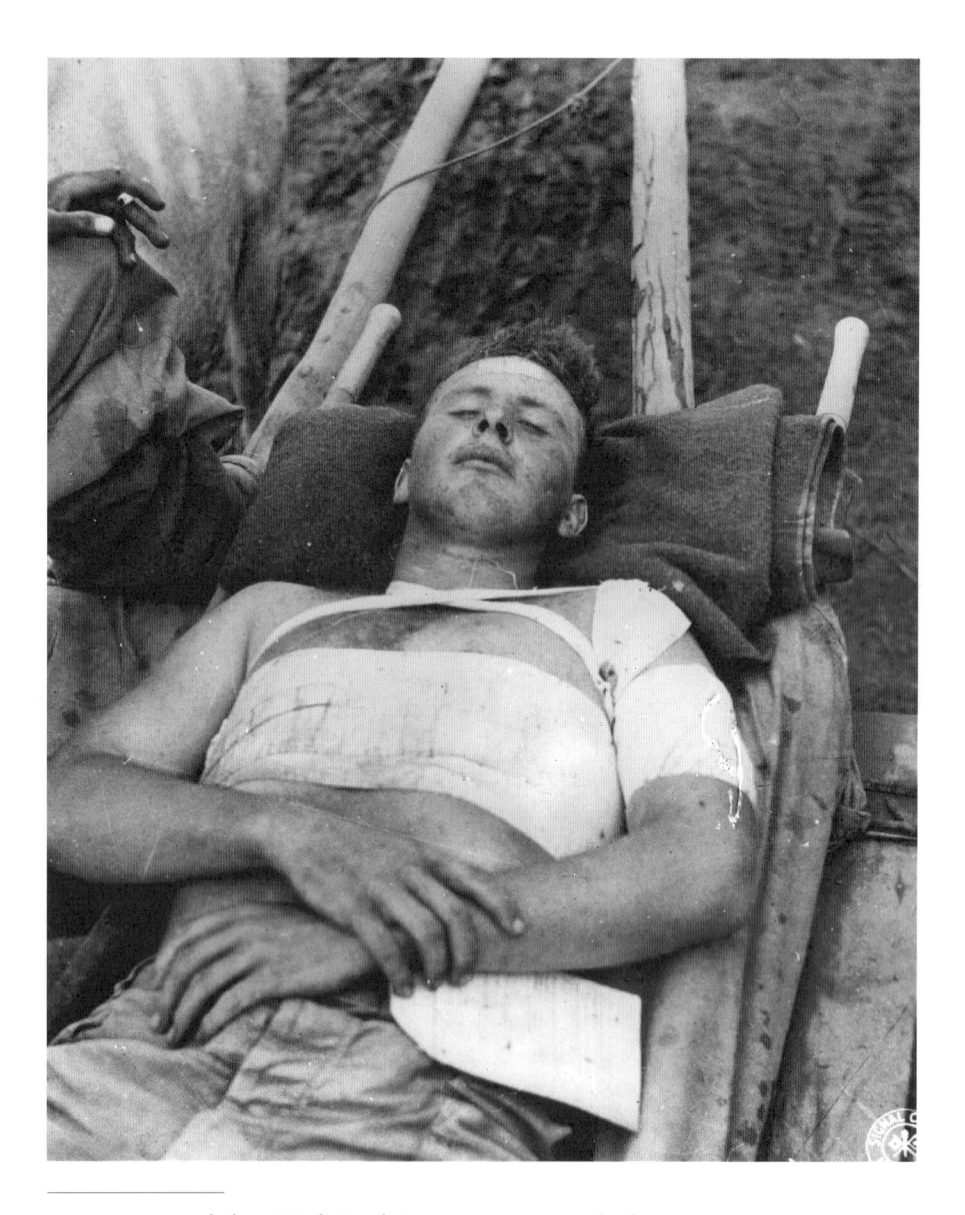

A private wounded at Myitkyina lying on an ox cart which would soon take him to a rescue plane.

一名在緬甸密支那受傷的士兵躺在牛車上,他很快會被送上前來接應的救援飛機。

Date of Photo 時間:不詳 N/A
Credits 來源:美國國家檔案館 Photo Courtesy of National Archives

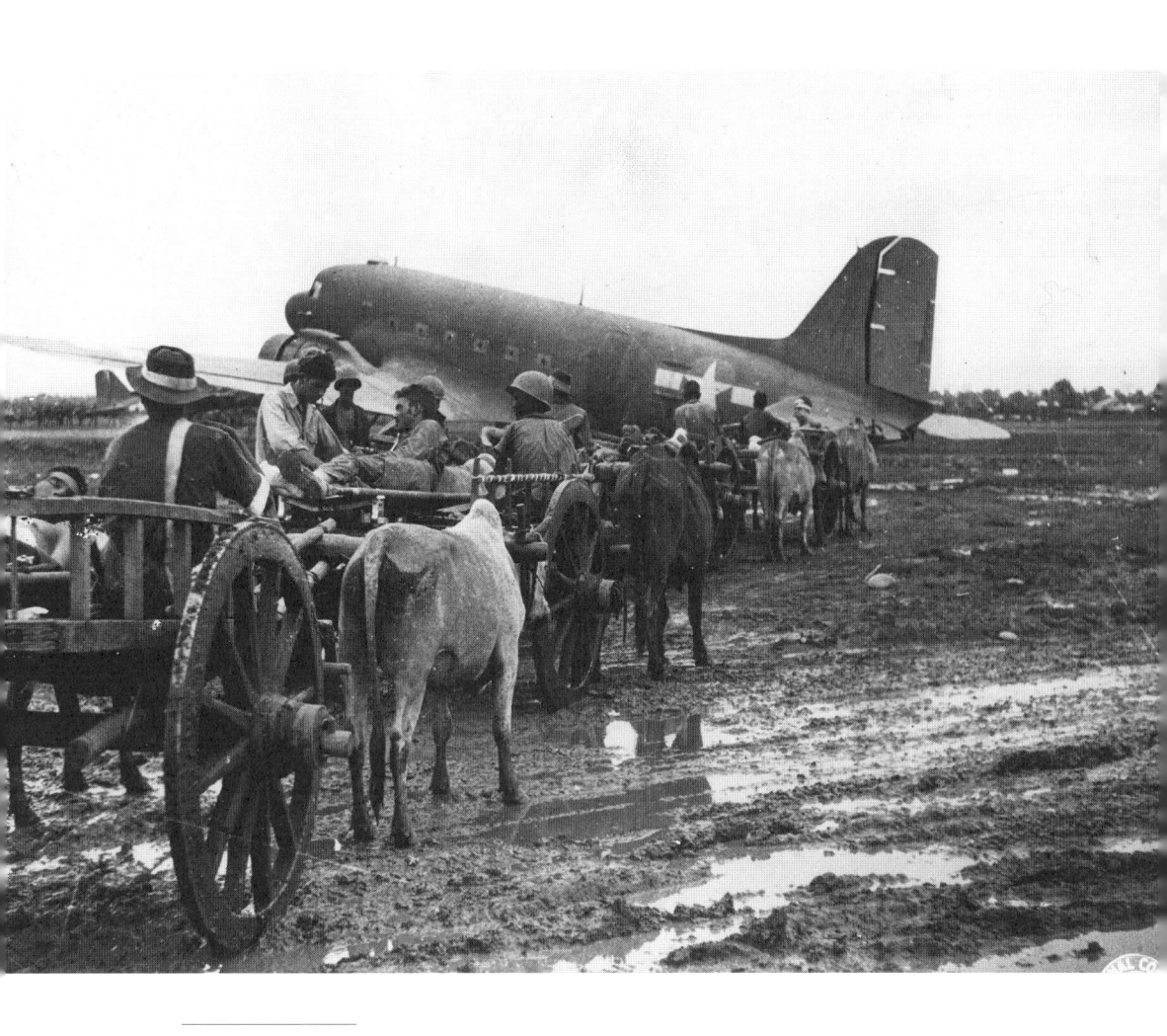

Oxen pulled wounded men from the Myitkyina front towards the waiting C-47 aircrafts.

牛車車隊將傷兵從密支那前線運送至待命中的 C-47 運輸機前。

Date of Photo 時間：不詳 N/A
Credits 來源：美國國家檔案館 Photo Courtesy of National Archives

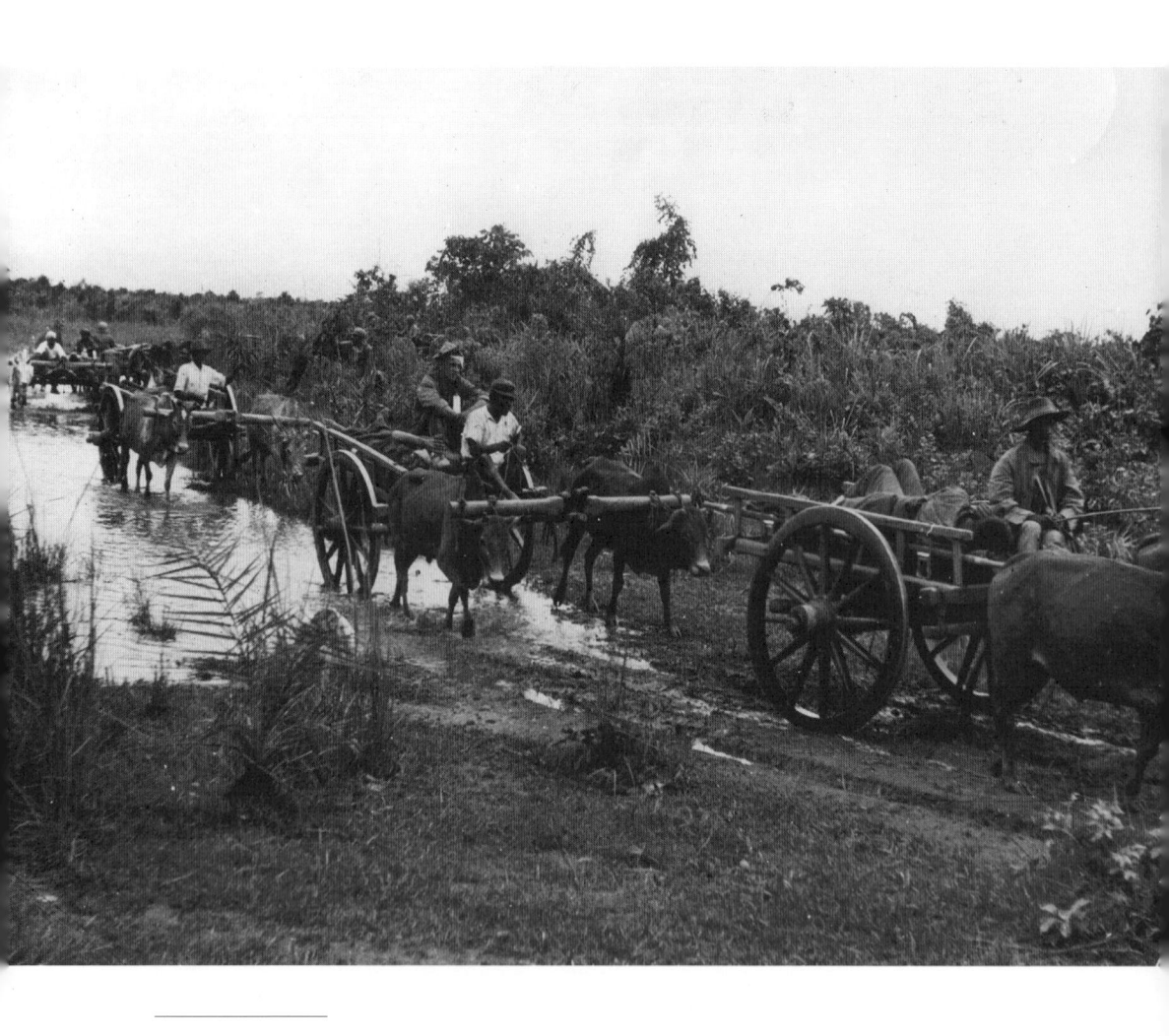

Oxen pulled wounded men from the Myitkyina front over five miles across muddy trails towards the air strip.

緬甸密支那前線的牛車車隊正拖運著傷兵,穿越五英里的泥濘小徑,前往機場跑道。

Date of Photo 時間:不詳 N/A
Credits 來源:美國國家檔案館 Photo Courtesy of National Archives

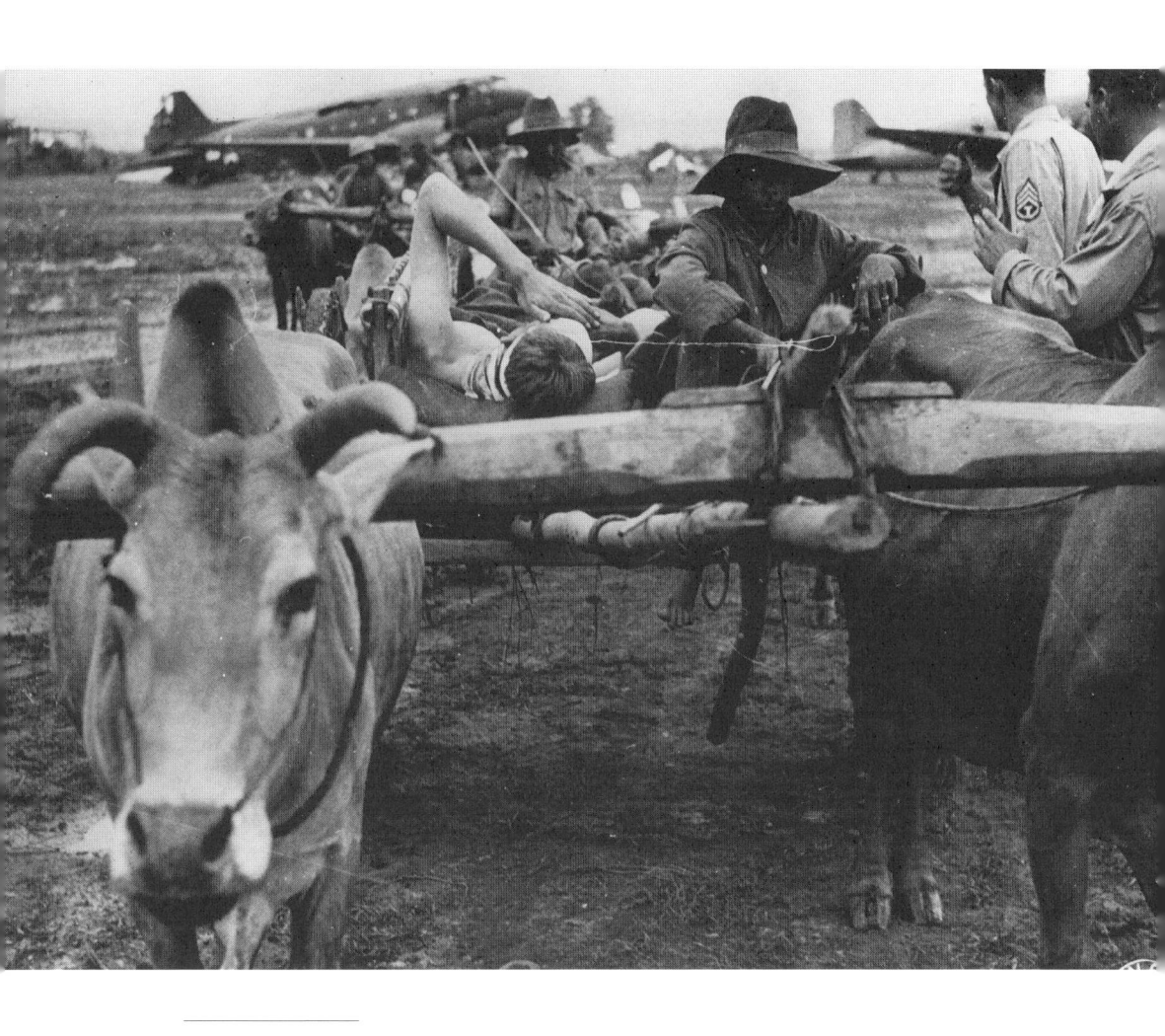

Wounded soldiers from Myitkyina laid on ox carts, lining up to be put into the waiting aircraft and transported to field hospitals.

來自緬甸密支那的傷兵躺在牛車上,排隊準備被抬上待命中的運輸機,轉送至野戰醫院。

Date of Photo 時間:不詳 N/A
Credits 來源:美國國家檔案館 Photo Courtesy of National Archives

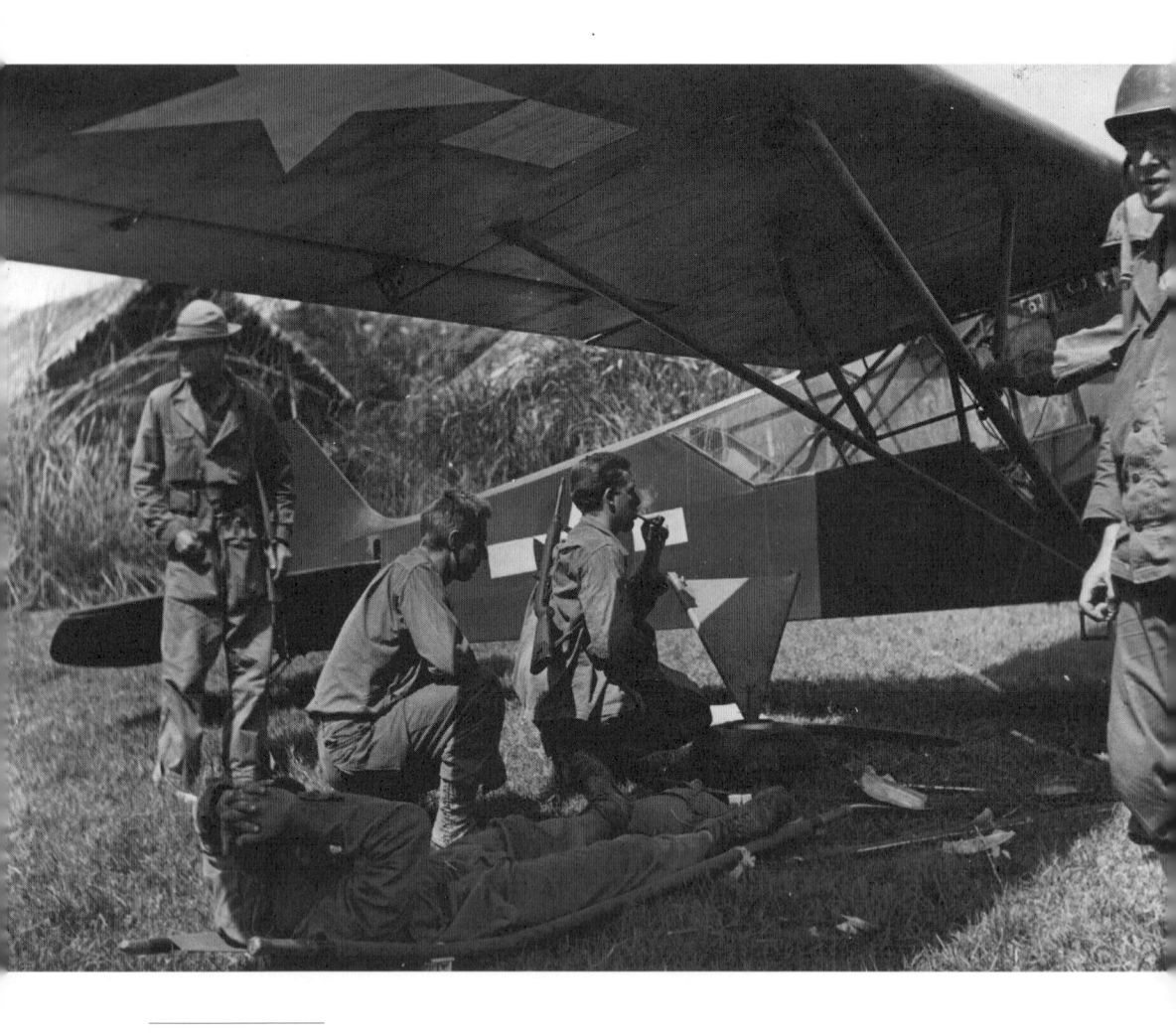

An American infantryman wounded in northern Burma was placed in a liaison plane and flown to a nearby hospital.

一名在緬甸北部受傷的美國步兵被安置在聯絡機中,緊急送往附近的醫院。

Date of Photo 時間:March 19, 1944
Credits 來源:美國國家檔案館 Photo Courtesy of National Archives

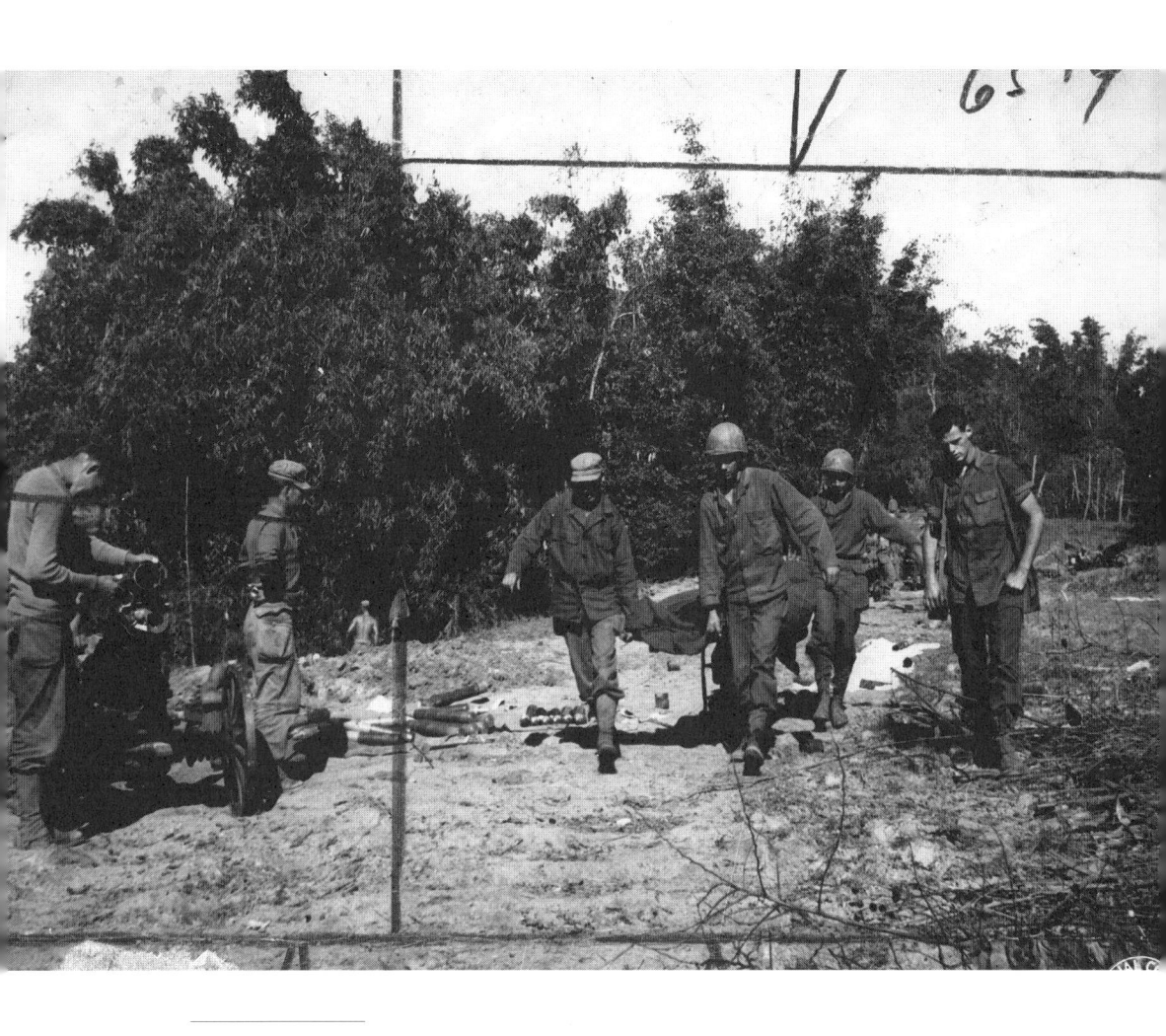

Wounded American soldiers on stretchers were carried to a first-aid station in Burma.

受傷的美國士兵躺在擔架上,被抬往緬甸的一處急救站。

Date of Photo 時間:January 28, 1945
Credits 來源:美國國家檔案館 Photo Courtesy of National Archives

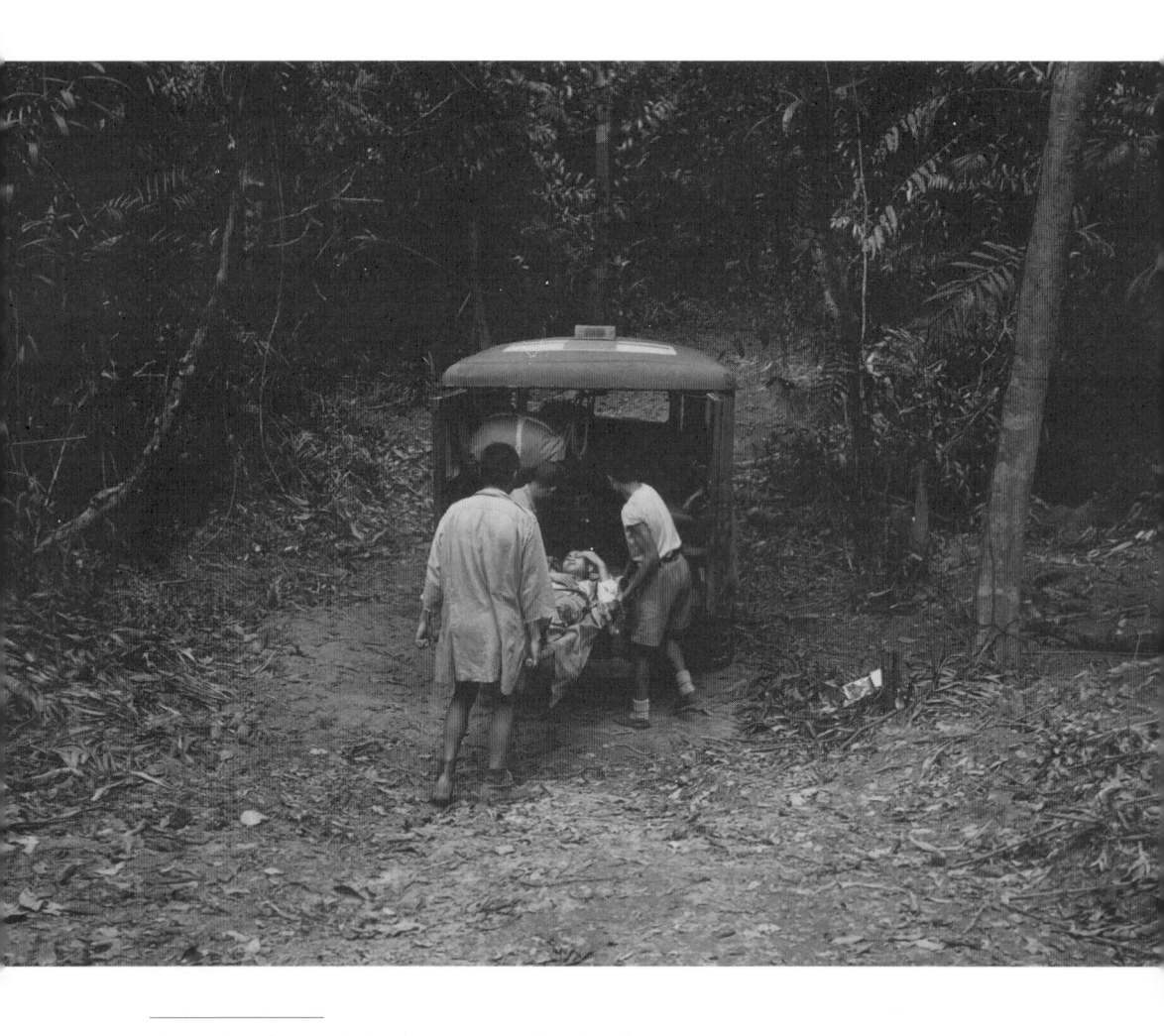

A casualty being loaded onto an WC-54 ambulance in Northern Burma.

在緬甸北部,一名傷患正被抬上 WC-54 救護車。

Date of Photo 時間:May 15, 1944
Credits 來源:美國國家檔案館 Photo Courtesy of National Archives

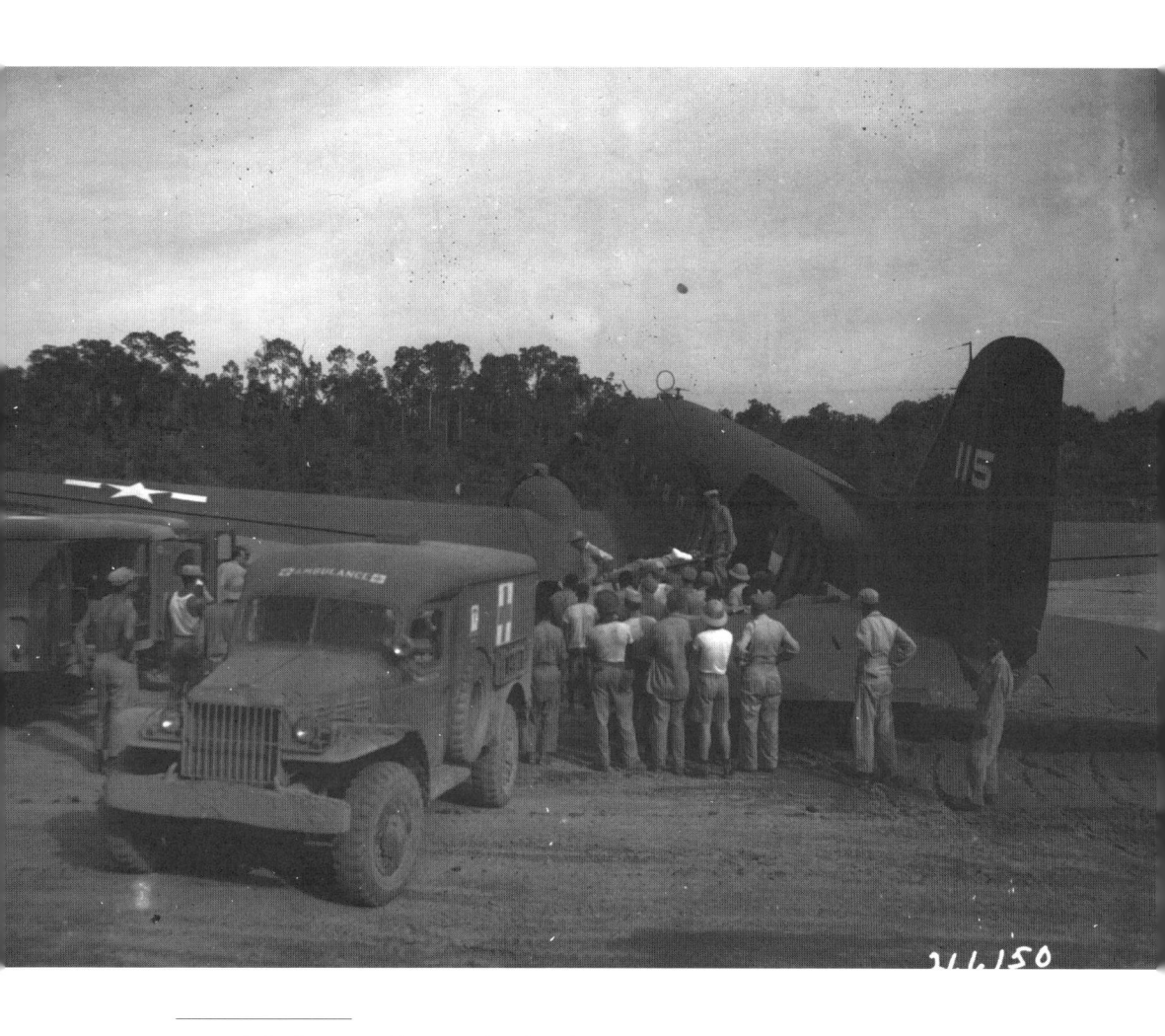

Wounded Chinese soldiers at the Shingbwiyang Airstrip in Northern Burma being unloaded from C-47 aircrafts onto WC-54 ambulances, which took them to the US Army's 73rd Evacuation Hospital.

在緬甸北部的欣貝延機場，幾位受傷的中國士兵從 C-47 運輸機上被抬下，轉移到 WC-54 救護車上，並由美軍送往第 73 後送醫院接受治療。

Date of Photo 時間：May 19, 1944
Credits 來源：美國國家檔案館 Photo Courtesy of National Archives

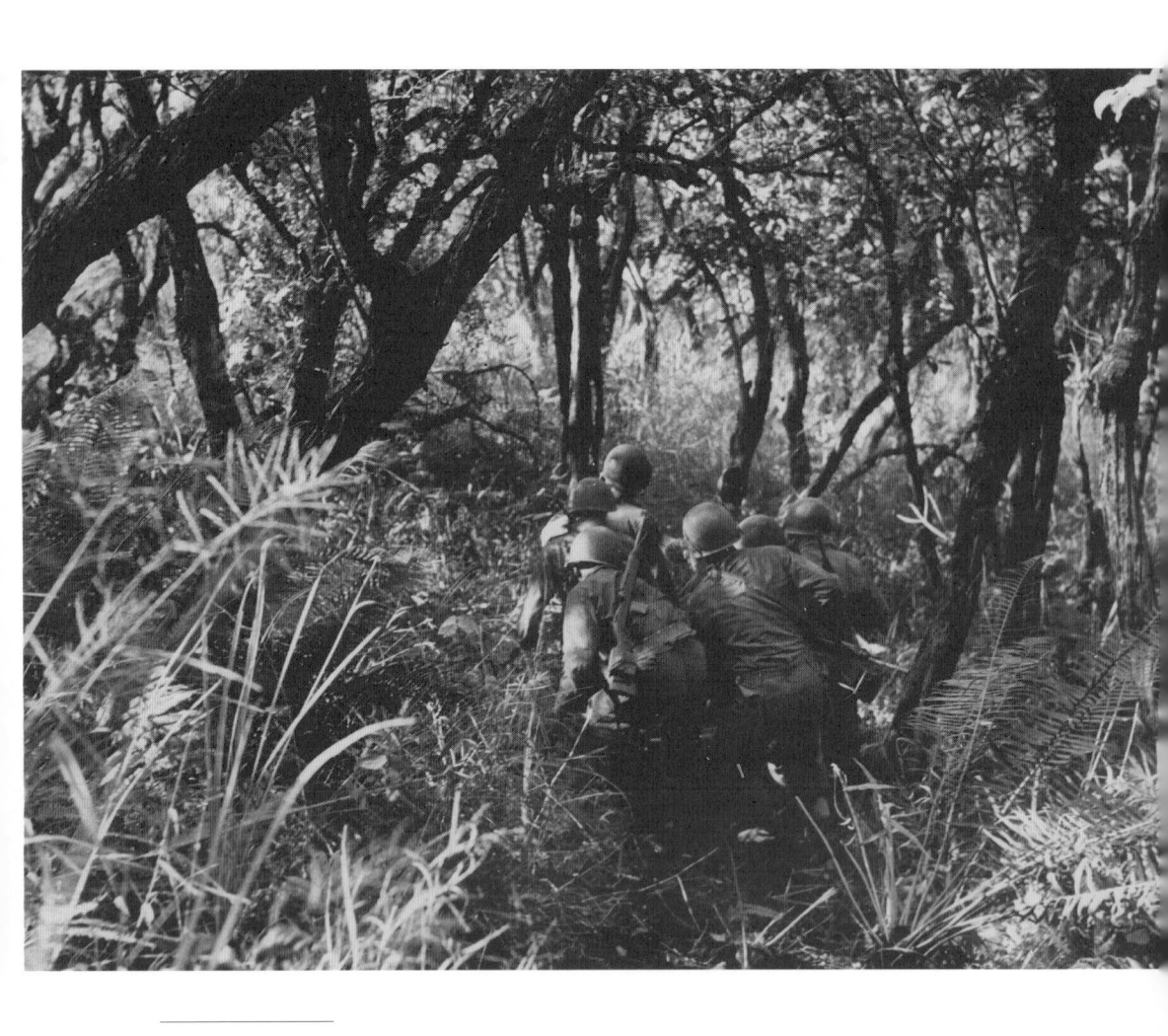

Soldiers of the US Army MARS Task Force long range penetration unit in Burma carrying their injured infantryman up to the aid station on a stretcher.

美軍步兵 5332 旅（代號「火星特遣隊」）深入緬甸作戰，多名步兵正用擔架抬著一位同袍前往救護站。

Date of Photo 時間：不詳 N/A
Credits 來源：美國國家檔案館 Photo Courtesy of National Archives

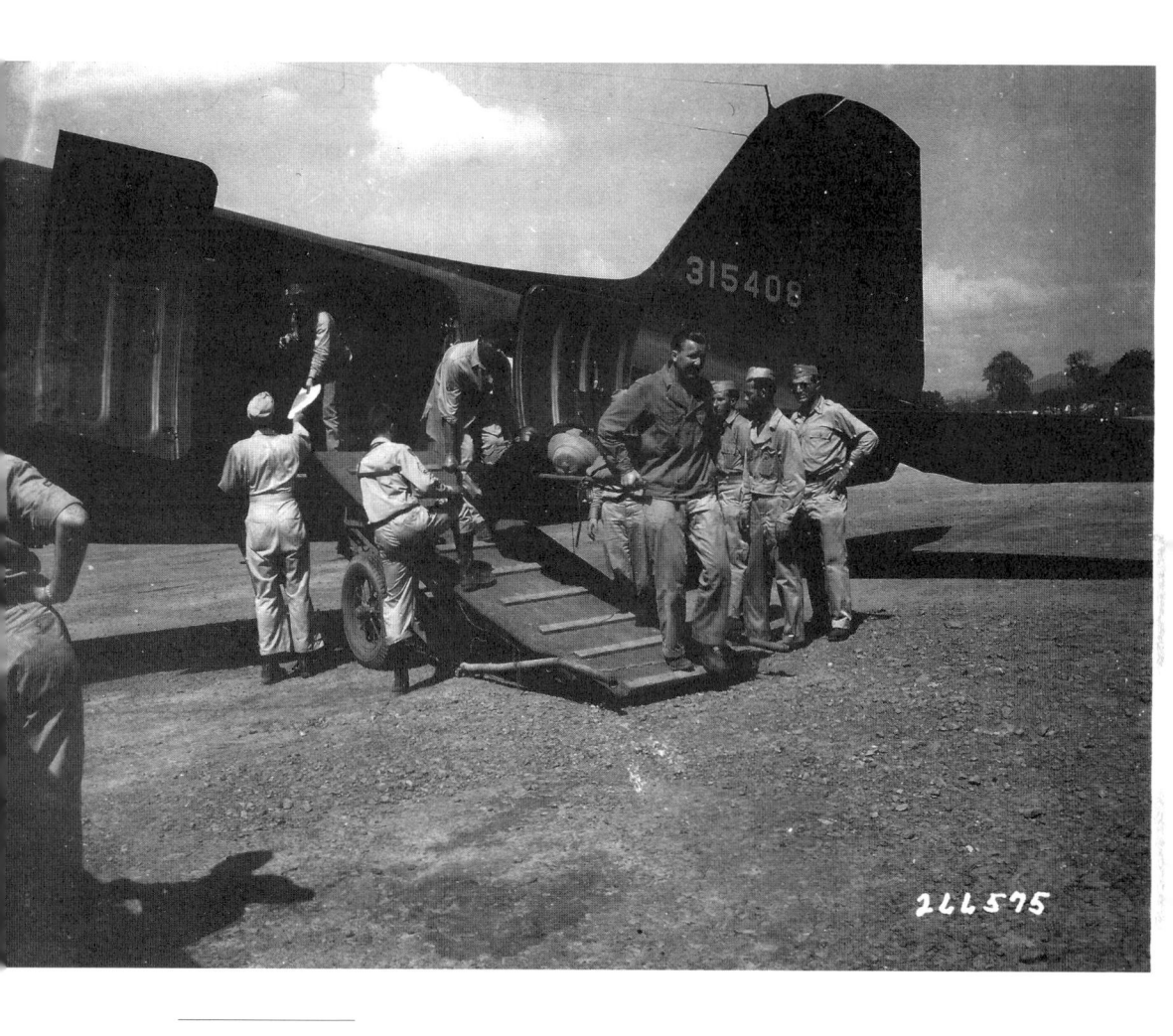

Wounded soldiers being removed from C-47 aircraft and transferred to a local field hospital.

美軍人員將傷兵從 C-47 運輸機上抬下，轉送至當地的野戰醫院接受治療。

Date of Photo 時間：May 19, 1944
Credits 來源：美國國家檔案館 Photo Courtesy of National Archives

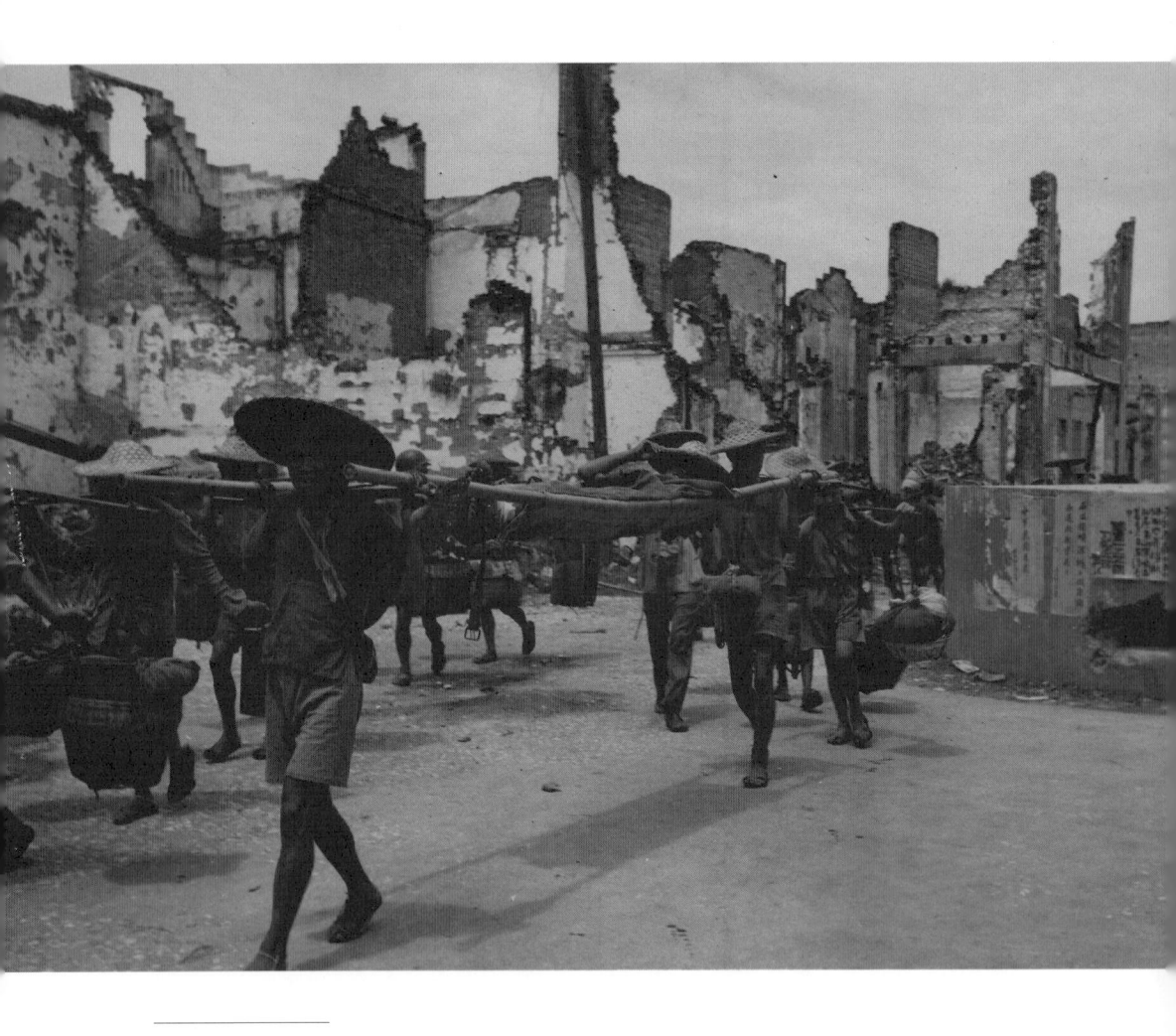

In Guilin, wounded Chinese were carried to the portable field hospital set up by the US Army Chinese Combat Command.

在桂林,一位受傷的中國人被抬往由美軍中國戰區作戰司令部設立的移動式野戰醫院接受治療。

Date of Photo 時間:不詳 N/A
Credits 來源:美國國家檔案館 Photo Courtesy of National Archives

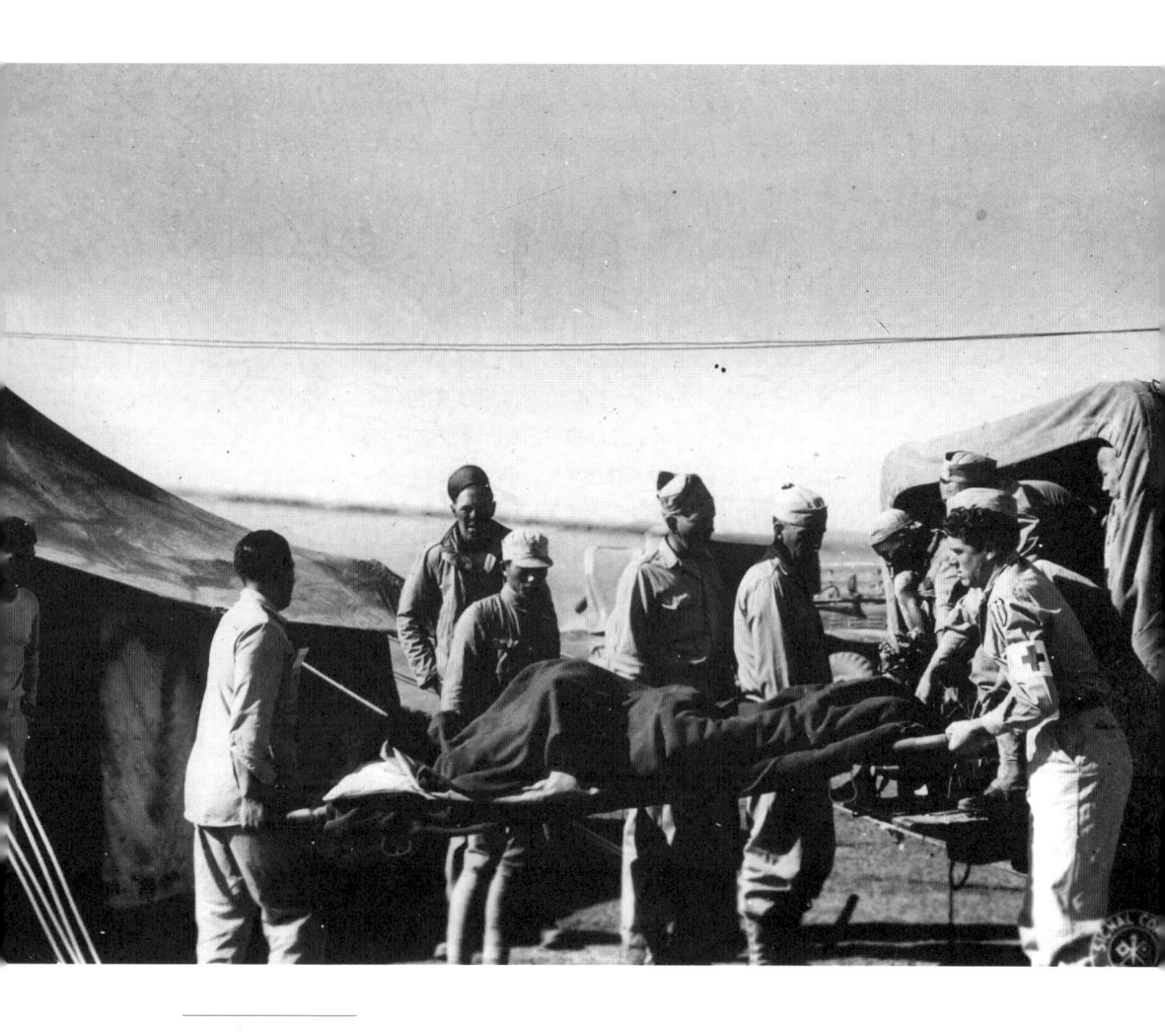

A wounded soldier being transferred from an ambulance to the receiving medical tent.

一名受傷士兵正從救護車下來,要到醫療帳篷接受治療。

Date of Photo 時間:February 28, 1945
Credits 來源:美國國家檔案館 Photo Courtesy of National Archives

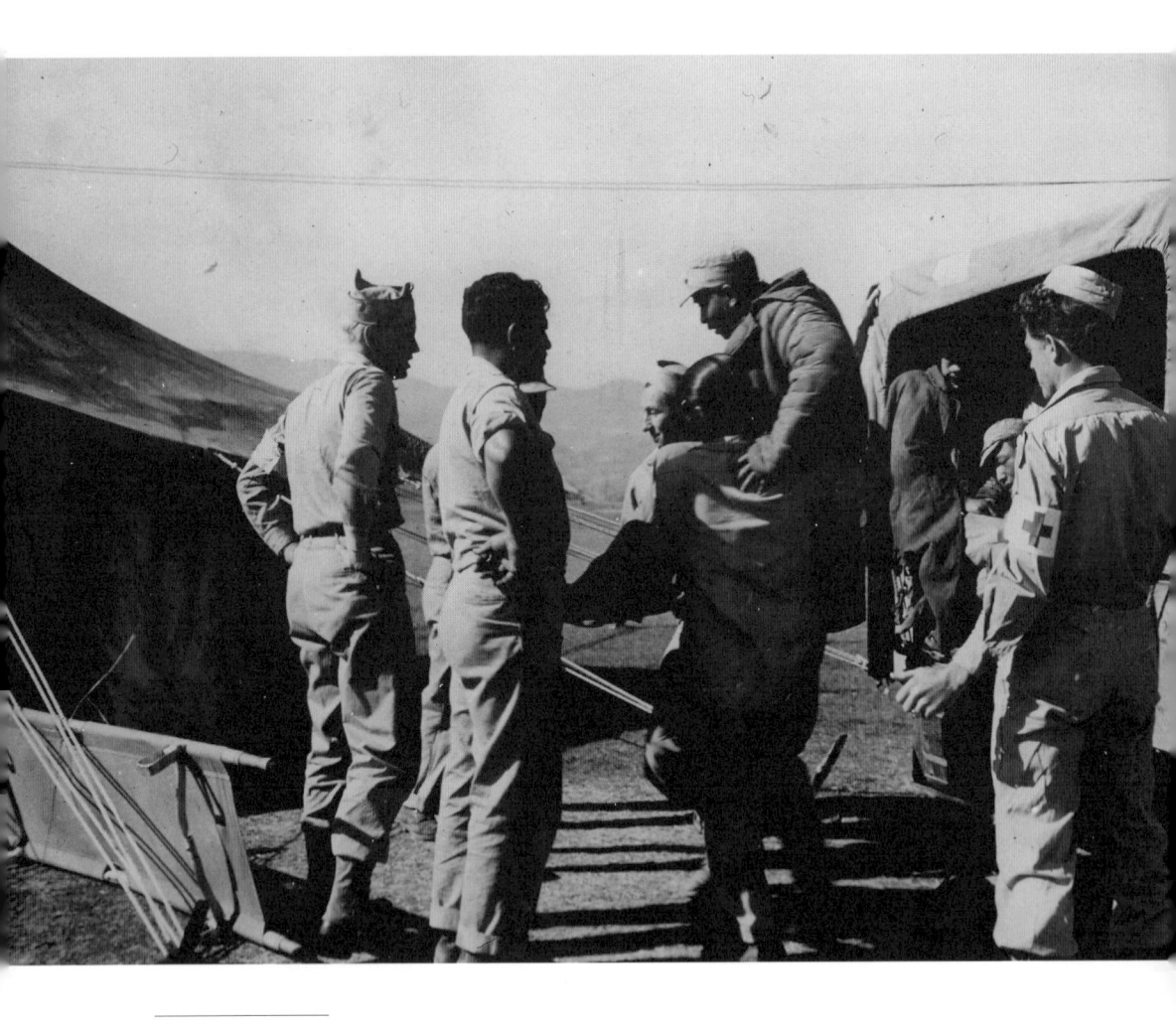

A wounded soldier being transferred from an ambulance to the receiving medical tent.

一名受傷士兵正從救護車下來，要到醫療帳篷接受治療。

Date of Photo 時間：February 28, 1945
Credits 來源：美國國家檔案館 Photo Courtesy of National Archives

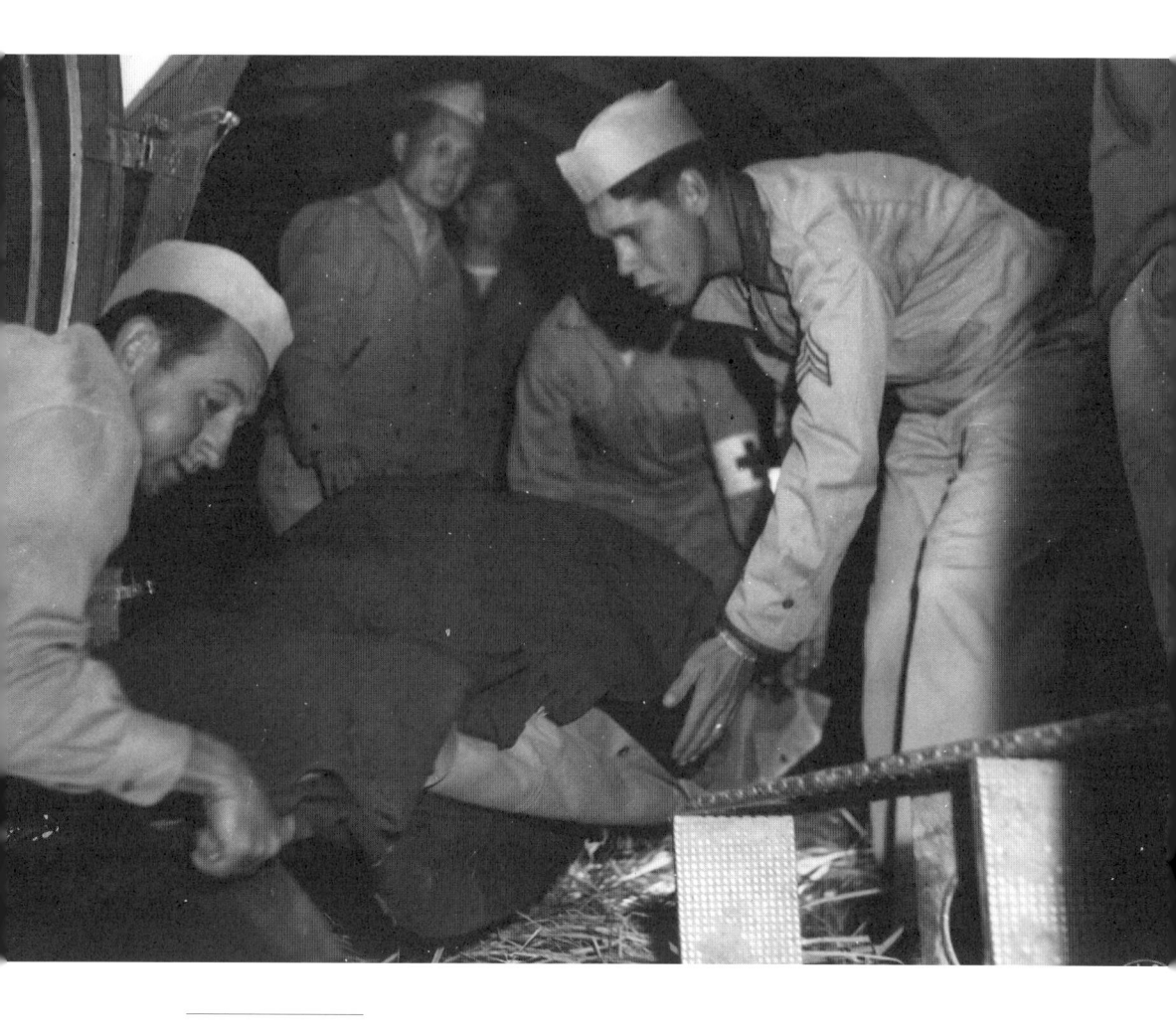

A patient being ushered from a C-47 to an ambulance after combat in Wanting.

在滇西畹町鎮的戰役後,一名傷患從 C-47 運輸機上被送上救護車,以便進一步治療。

Date of Photo 時間:不詳 N/A
Credits 來源:美國國家檔案館 Photo Courtesy of National Archives

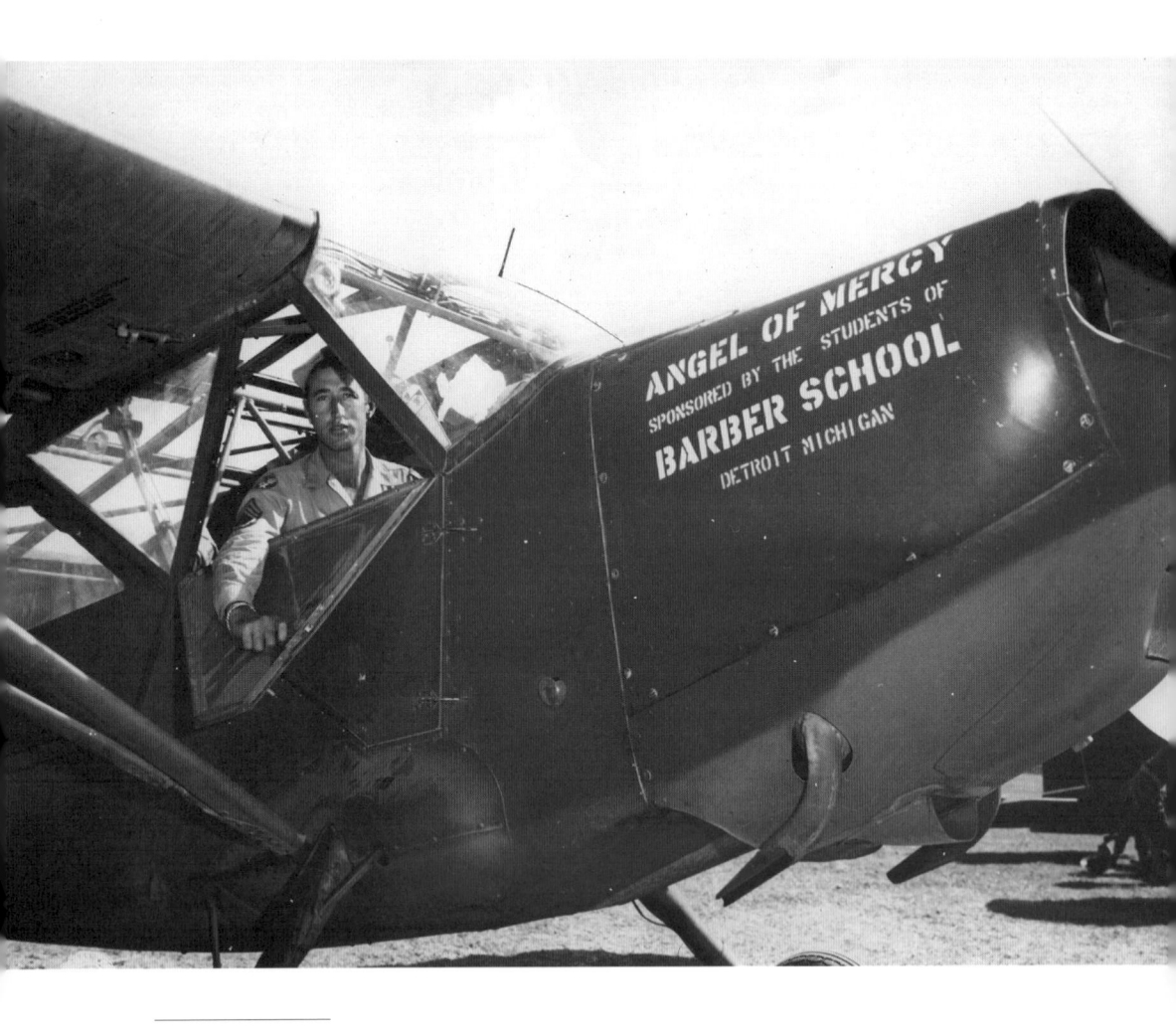

An American pilot looking out of an L-5 Liaison plane. The plane in question was donated by Barber School in Detroit, Michigan.

一位美國飛行員從一架 L-5 聯絡機內向外眺望。這架飛機是由密西根州底特律市的巴伯學校（Barber School）捐贈。

Date of Photo 時間：February 17, 1945
Credits 來源：美國國家檔案館 Photo Courtesy of National Archives

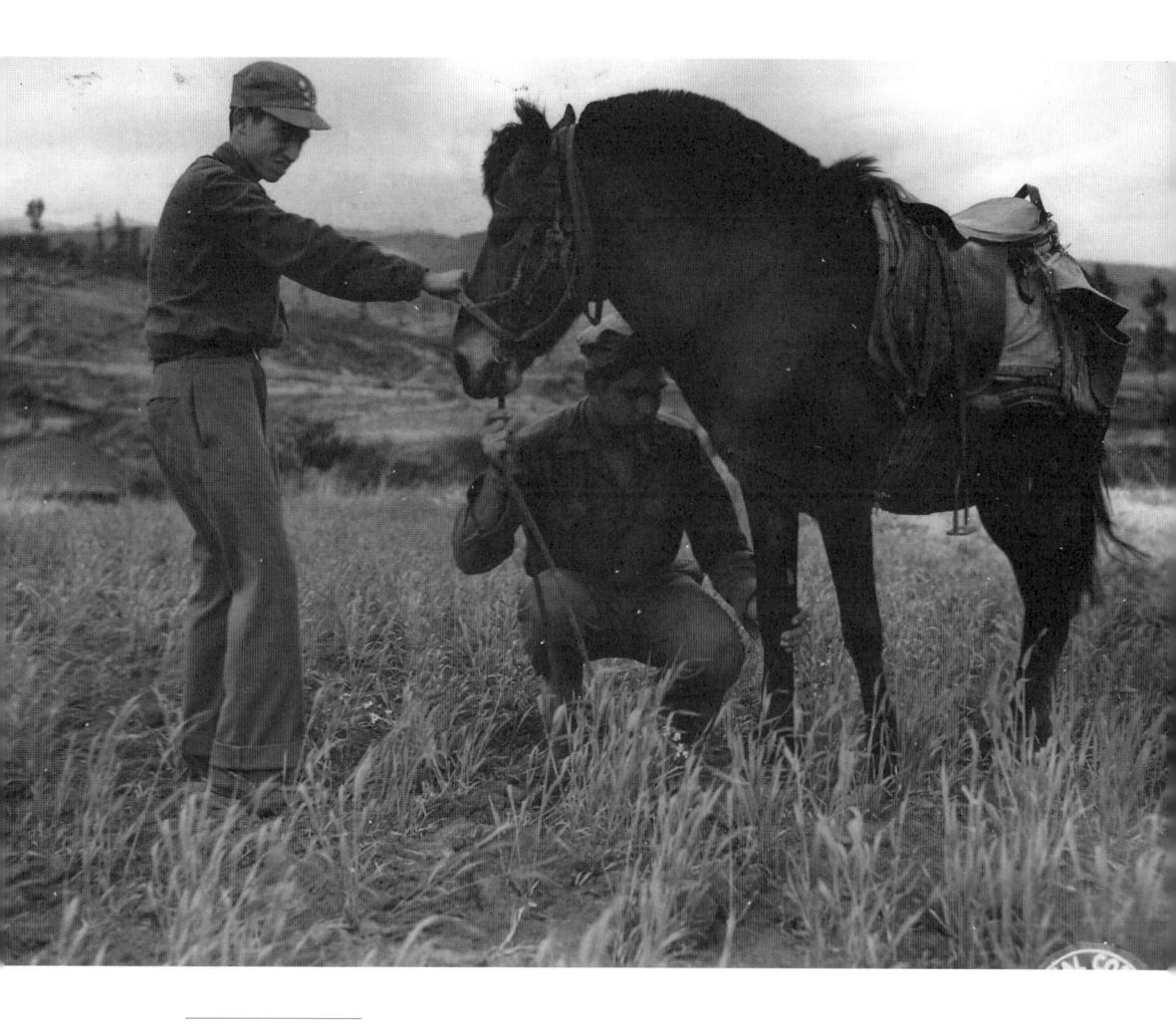

Two Chinese soldiers examining a horse for lameness.

兩名中國士兵正在檢查這匹馬是否跛腳。

Date of Photo 時間：February 1, 1946
Credits 來源：美國國家檔案館 Photo Courtesy of National Archives

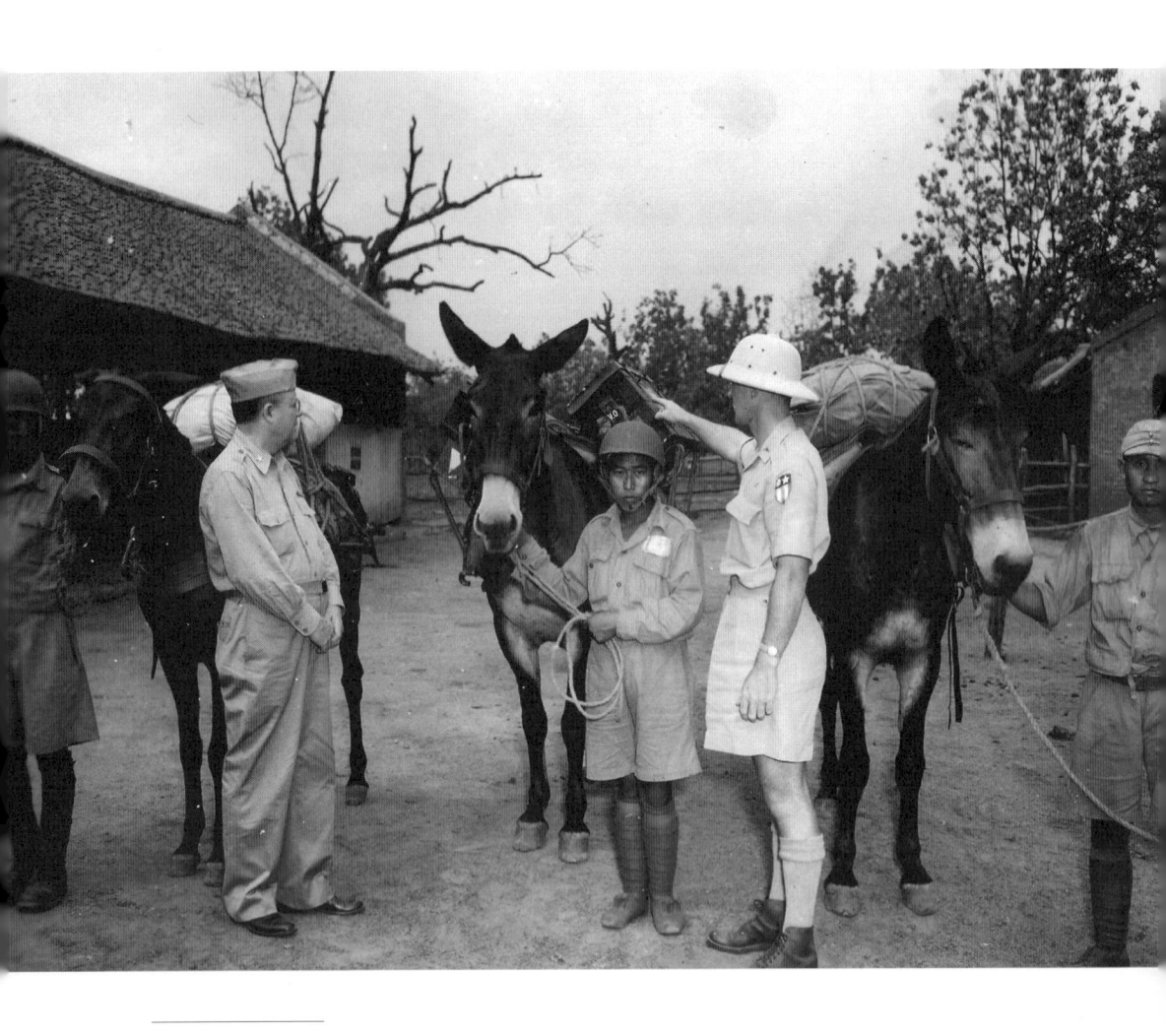

Forces in India transporting medical supplies via mule pack trains.
駐紮在印度的部隊利用騾子運輸隊運送醫療物資。

Date of Photo 時間：October 16, 1944
Credits 來源：美國國家檔案館 Photo Courtesy of National Archives

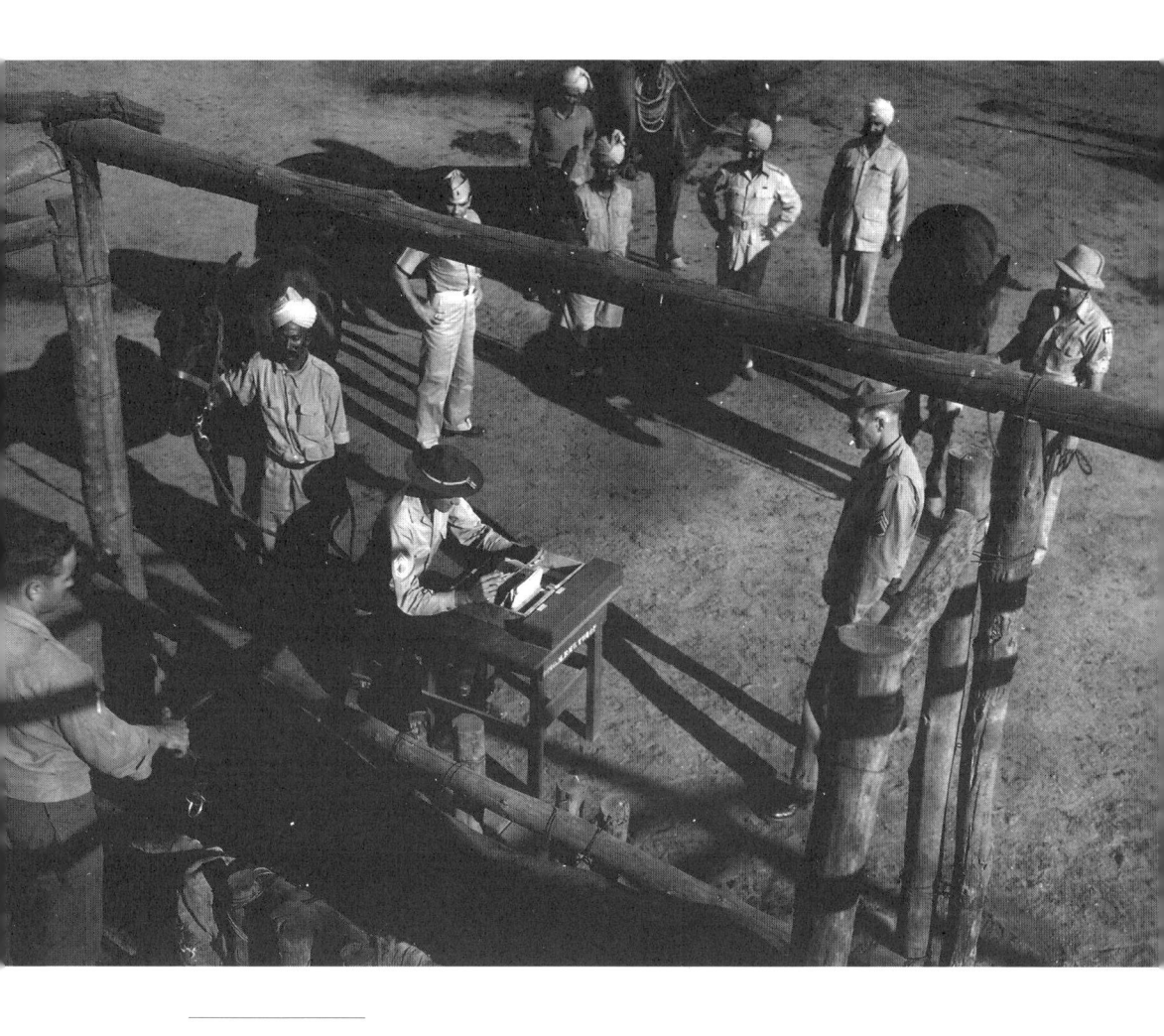

A quartermaster inspecting the veterinary records of their troop's pack mules.

一名軍需官正在檢查部隊馱獸的獸醫紀錄。

Date of Photo 時間：November 24, 1944
Credits 來源：美國國家檔案館 Photo Courtesy of National Archives

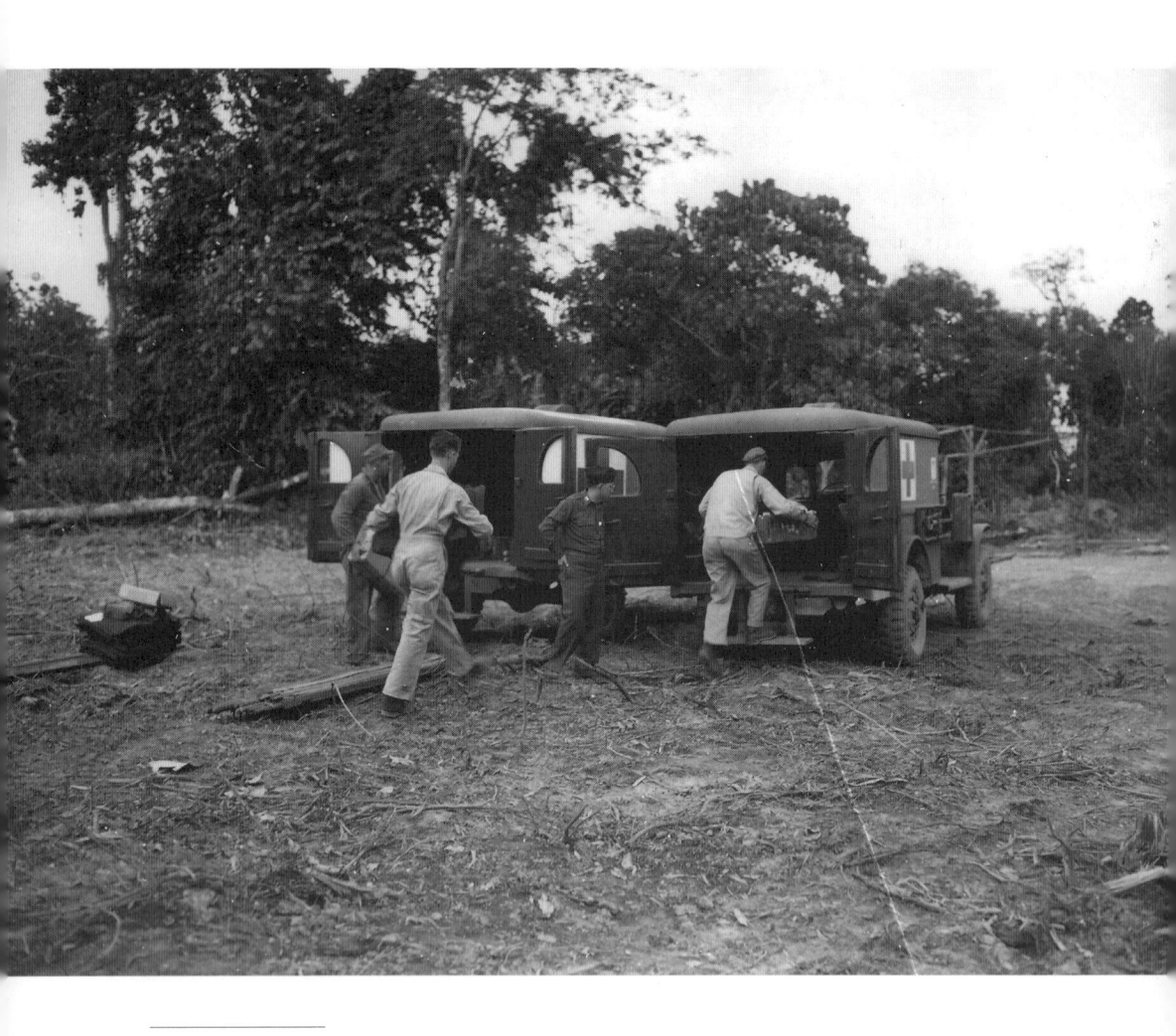

Troops loaded up two ambulances, which would accompany the First Corps journey from India to China.

部隊裝載了兩輛救護車的物資,即將要跟著第一軍從印度前往中國。

Date of Photo 時間:March 19, 1945
Credits 來源:美國國家檔案館 Photo Courtesy of National Archives

OPERATIONS AND ADVANCEMENTS

With the relocation of the Guomindang Nationalist Party to Chongqing in November 1937, primary medical operations during the Second Sino-Japanese War were carried out in southwestern China. The provision of vaccine samples, penicillin production technology, blood banks, and medical supplies from the United States government and private organizations not only saved countless Chinese lives and sustained both military and civilian populations but also strengthened the Chinese military's resistance against Japanese forces. The training of Chinese medical personnel, along with humanitarian aid and joint medical operations, contributed to the development of China's medical infrastructure and laid the foundation for modern medical practices in China.

Military-Medical Collaboration

In the autumn of 1942, many physicians from the International Medical Relief Corps (IMRC) left Tuyunguan to join the Chinese Expeditionary Force-X in India and Burma. Each division included three officers and two doctors. Those who stayed in China continued to serve with Dr. Robert Lin on the southern front in Yunnan Province as part of the Chinese Expeditionary Force-Y, based in Kunming.

In 1943, the Chinese Red Cross deployed twenty-four surgical teams with the Chinese army in Yunnan, including three foreign teams from Friends Ambulance Units and the British Red Cross. Under Allied command, the United States military, the International Relief Committee, the Chinese Red Cross, and IMRC physicians coordinated efforts. In November 1944, the Chinese Training and Combat Command was established, integrating Y-Force and Z-Force operations to train and support Chinese forces in Central and Southern China.

Qualified Chinese medical personnel were scarce, as most skilled physicians remained in treaty ports like Hong Kong, Shanghai, and Guangzhou, unwilling to join the military. The United States Army in the China-Burma-India Theater filled gaps in the Chinese Army with trained medical personnel and enhanced military medical services by prioritizing life conservation. An American Medical Unit from the United States Army's Chinese Combat Command advanced with Chinese troops into Guilin, staffed by United States Army medical personnel providing efficient frontline care for the wounded. Utilizing the best medical knowledge and surgical techniques available in the United States, the unit significantly boosted Chinese troop morale. The presence of immediate medical aid reassured Chinese soldiers, fostering greater bravery in combat.

Upon the outbreak of the Second Sino-Japanese War, Dr. Robert Lin organized the first shipment of medical supplies to the battlefield and secured medical aid and international relief from the Chinese branch of the International Red Cross. Later, he led the Chinese Red Cross Medical Relief Corps (CRCMRC), headquartered in Tuyunguan, Guizhou Province, organizing medical teams, distributing supplies, and training personnel to manage emergencies. As chairman of the Army Medical Administration in the Nationalist government's Military Affairs Commission, and with donations from the American Bureau of Medical Aid to China (ABMAC), Dr. Robert Lin also established the Emergency Medical Service Training School (EMSTS) at Tuyunguan in 1938. Staffed by some of his former PUMC students and colleagues, the EMSTS trained nurses, stretcher-bearers, and field medical orderlies to provide immediate battlefield care. Meiyu Zhou (Měiyù Zhōu) a 1930 nursing graduate from PUMC, founded the Army School of Nursing at the EMSTS in Guiyang. Her efforts, along with those of other PUMC alumni, significantly advanced military nursing services and education in China during this tumultuous period.

The EMSTS collaborated with the ABMAC to integrate the dominant German structure of Chinese military medicine into American standards and trained over 13,000 medical personnel to respond to both military and civilian medical needs during the war. Its sanitary training programs engaged local helpers in public health services and helped establish several nursing schools for young women, and health centers in remote areas of China, which helped maintain modern healthcare systems during wartime. The school also organized a field ambulance battalion that was staffed with Army medical officers and Red Cross personnel, to train local helpers in coordinating supplies and personnel and improve the transportation of medical services.

The shortage of physicians remained critical in wartime China. By the end of 1941, the Chinese Red Cross Medical Relief Corps had only 181 doctors, including some foreign physician volunteers from the IMRC. In Yan'an, the Bethune International Peace Hospital of the Eighth Route Army had only nine physicians, while the Chinese Communist Party's New Fourth Army had fewer than sixty qualified physicians serving millions, and even tens of millions, of people. Graduates of the EMSTS joined the Army Sanitary Corps and the Red Cross Medical Relief Corps, serving on the frontlines and in unoccupied areas, where nurses and nursing orderlies trained at the EMSTS performed most of the medical treatment.

Blood Operations

Medical blood transfusion was essential for surgical operations, emergency care, and certain disease treatments, however, it required a blood bank to ensure a regular blood supply, especially during the harrowing wartime. With ABMAC's support, two Chinese doctors went to study blood plasma production under Dr. John Scudder at Columbia University. One of them received further training at Bryn Mawr Hospital. A Chinese American bacteriologist from the University of Wisconsin joined the project. ABMAC also enlisted 817 blood donors of diverse racial backgrounds in the United States, who viewed their contributions as aiding China's military modernization and the war effort. The collected blood was then processed into plasma and shipped to China.

Through the efforts of Dr. Robert Lin and donations from ABMAC, China's first blood bank was established in Kunming in 1943, equipped with state-of-the-art technology for preparing freeze-dried plasma. This development significantly strengthened China's wartime medical relief efforts. During the intense Tengchong combat in Yunnan in the autumn of 1944, a military surgeon reported that nearly all wounded soldiers who received plasma transfusions had very fortunately survived.

However, a challenge arose as traditional Chinese beliefs viewed blood as integral to the body, associating blood loss with diminished vitality and a disregard for the parental gift of life. This cultural perception made blood donations, both for blood banks and for general medical care, rare, especially among soldiers who feared that donating blood would weaken them. Only a small segment of urban elites who had been exposed to Western medicine understood and accepted the practice of blood donation.

To emphasize its military role in supplying blood to Chinese soldiers, ABMAC and Dr. Robert Lin named the facility the Blood Storage Unit of the Army Medical Administration. Despite support from Chinese military leaders, initial efforts to secure blood donations were hampered by soldiers' reluctance, widespread malnutrition, unsanitary conditions, and poor communication. In addition, unreliable electricity and water supplies hindered the operation of essential equipment like autoclaves, centrifuges, and refrigerators. Hand-operated pumps and the conversion of machines to charcoal power further limited the blood bank's capacity to process donations. A contaminated plasma incident delayed operations for months as the blood bank implemented new sterilization methods and equipment to restore donor confidence.

To further improve low donor turnout, doctors, nurses, and assistants of blood bank mobile units traveled to army camps, schools, and labor sites to collect blood. This initiative significantly boosted donations, accounting for 92% of all collected blood by the end of the war in 1945. Additionally, the blood bank launched campaigns appealing to civilians' sense of altruism and nationalism, while offering essential food items as rewards. College students from National Southwest Associated University (Xinan Lianda) and workers from electric and railroad companies enthusiastically participated, securing vital civilian blood donations during wartime China.

Battlefield Surgical Operations

The India-Burma and China Theaters relied entirely on air transportation over the Himalayan Hump for logistical support. Malaria spread rapidly, but medicines were scarce. Battlefields in mountains, jungles, and valleys, combined with monsoon rains, made motor transportation impractical. Medical equipment such as X-rays and microscopes were unavailable in combat zones under enemy fire, as these had to be carried on soldiers' backs, transported by pack animals, or dropped by parachute. As a result, battlefield surgeries were performed in portable surgical units or hospitals that were set up in temporary structures like tents or requisitioned buildings to provide immediate surgical care near the front lines. In the eastern China combat area, there were only four portable surgical hospitals, each unit staffed by two surgeons and eighteen corpsmen. Corpsmen were responsible for undressing patients, cleaning wounds, performing superficial debridement, and administering intravenous anesthesia when necessary. Surgeons moved quickly from one patient to another along the line of tables, suturing superficial wounds, enucleating eyes, or amputating a leg or an arm as required.

In May 1945, Colonels Benjamin J. Birk, a surgeon of the Chinese Combat Command, and other consultants traveled to Zijiang, the most forward fighter base after the fall of Guilin to fierce Japanese attacks, and Anjiang, the headquarters of the Eastern Command within the Chinese Combat Command. They inspected Chinese and United States Army hospitals, recognizing the high quality of surgery performed under immense pressure and the excellent service of the medical teams despite a significant backlog of patients awaiting operations.

Vaccination

The China National Epidemic Prevention Bureau (NEPB) was established in 1919 to manufacture vaccines and sera to control a local plague outbreak in northern China. When the full-scale Sino-Japanese War escalated in 1937, the shortage of medicine and medical supplies, lack of health infrastructure and sanitation, poor living conditions, malnutrition, and the wartime migrations of soldiers and refugees led to devastating outbreaks of cholera in crowded cities and refugee camps, and malaria and bacterial dysentery among Chinese troops. Vaccination remained a top priority for the China National Health Administration.

With support from international aid organizations such as the State Serum Institute of Denmark, the American National Institutes of Health, and the British Medical Research Council, and particularly the League of Nations, the NEPB imported standard vaccine samples and equipment. They reestablished biochemical laboratories in Kunming, Guiyang, and Lanzhou. Between 1937 and 1945, they produced millions of doses of vaccines against smallpox, cholera, typhoid fever, and other diseases using experimental animals. The Chinese Red Cross also developed its own vaccine production facility in Guiyang, producing six million doses annually by 1943 for cholera, typhoid, diphtheria, tetanus, and typhus.

In 1941, the Chinese government broadcasted that immunization was a crucial weapon against potential Japanese biological warfare and mandated preventive vaccinations against cholera, dysentery, and typhoid for officers and soldiers at the front and civilians at the rear. While vaccination efforts reduced the severity and occurrence of epidemics, Japanese air raids, shipment delays, contamination, expiration, inadequate health infrastructure, and public resistance to vaccination challenged mass immunization efforts during the war.

Penicillin

Kunming was the center of U.S. Army Air Forces air transport in China. Due to the location advantage, NEPB staff accessed newly published foreign scholarly journals, such as The Lancet, and received news of penicillin's successful therapeutic development in the West. In the spring of 1944, two NEPB staff members traveled to India with support from the Rockefeller Foundation to survey public health organizations there, returning to China with ten strains of penicillin that had been isolated in England and America. Then, a Chinese microbiologist returning from the University of Wisconsin brought an additional three strains. The NEPB also obtained strains of penicillin from the United States Northern Regional Research Laboratory in Peoria, Illinois, where researchers had developed fermentation methods to culture penicillin within. NEPB staff sought means of cultivating and purifying the strains.

The ABMAC worked with the China National Health Administration and the Chinese Red Cross to allocate funds for the purchase of medical supplies and equipment from the United States. Unable to purchase penicillin directly for distribution in China, ABMAC established a small plant in New York jointly with American Committee in Aid of Chinese Industrial Cooperatives (Indusco) trying to provide China not only a method for producing penicillin but also a technique for research on and production of antibiotic substances in China.

The plant developed methods of producing crude and refined penicillin using only materials and equipment available in the basic conditions of wartime China. It trained a Chinese bacteriologist who had received a PhD from Johns Hopkins University in methods of penicillin production and returned to China, taking charge of training personnel and establishing new production laboratories in the unoccupied territory in China.

Due to technical problems, NEPB failed to produce penicillin. The ABMAC invited American bacteriologists to discuss the technical problems of cultivating penicillin in wartime China and identified the unavailability of corn steep liquor, the crucial additive for culture mediums. With the material and funds of about nineteen million Chinese Yuan from ABMAC in support of the penicillin production, and through numerous experiments on substitutes, the NEPB managed to produce five ampoules of penicillin, each containing five thousand Oxford units in September 1944. In August 1944, as a result of the Lend-Lease Act, the United States Army Air Forces transported 465 ampoules containing 46.5 million units of penicillin penicillin to Chinese hospitals. Penicillin and sulfa drugs became available to treat battlefield infections in wartime China in 1944.

Dental Care

Beijing Union Medical College maintained a Department of Dentistry, contributing to the training of dental professionals and the promotion of modern dental practices in wartime China. During the Second Sino-Japanese War, China's dental care infrastructure was destroyed. Some international dentists such as

Russian dentist Dimitri Afonsky, and the United States Army Dental Corps in China provided dental care, dental surgeons, and dental education to Chinese military personnel. The United States Army Dental Corps provided dental care to American and Allied troops and expanded to the China Theater, formerly part of CBI Theater. As the China Theater dental surgeon, Lieutenant Colonel Richard D. Darby oversaw dental services across the vast and logistically challenging China Theater, including transporting dental supplies over the treacherous "Hump" from India to China.

The equipment, instruments, and supplies in the Medical Department were used for general dental operative work in the field hospitals. A dental prosthetic laboratory was established in early 1944, despite significant equipment and supply shortages. An acetylene generator had to be built to ensure the laboratory had a supply of gas and carbide gas was installed late in 1944. This laboratory, with only two dental officers and seven enlisted men, produced full and partial dentures, repaired dental prosthetics, and fabricated bridges to address the dental needs of Chinese military personnel. In addition, mobile dental clinics were set up in tents or repurposed structures, enabling dental teams to provide essential care, including extractions, restorations, and emergency treatments, often near front-line areas.

Recognizing the lack of dental care within the Chinese Army, United States Army Dental Corps officers initiated the first dental training program in China for the Chinese Medical and Pharmacy Corps officers. The first one-month course commenced in November 1943 in Dali, Yunnan Province, focusing on the fundamentals of oral surgery and the treatment of oral diseases. Considering the travel challenges for the students to travel as many as twenty days to reach the school in Dali, United States Army Dental Corps instructors travel to the various Chinese divisions to conduct condensed courses to equip Chinese units with basic dental care capabilities.

In April 1944, the United States Army Dental Corps opened another dental training school in Guilin, China with the number of students limited to twelve. Two female nurses in the Chinese Army with the rank of second and first lieutenant took the course. As of July 25, 1944, when the school was forced to close due to Japanese fierce attacks, a total of twenty-four students of two classes graduated and twelve more students in the process were trained in part from the dental training school in Guilin.

Psychiatric Support

Poverty, disease, natural disasters, and immense war devastation had lasting traumatic impacts on Chinese survivors. Psychiatric support in wartime China was necessary but limited due to the war focus on physical health, cultural stigma around mental health, and lack of trained professionals. In the late 19th and early 20th centuries, Western medical missionaries and physicians were among the first to introduce Western psychiatric practices in China. American medical missionary and philanthropist John G. Kerr helped establish the Canton Hospital for the Insane, China's first modern facility for mental health care in 1898 in Guangzhou. Austrian neuropsychiatrist Fanny Halpern collaborated with local elites and opened Shanghai Mercy Hospital, the first psychiatric hospital in Shanghai.

Influenced by American models, the Guomindang government converted the existing Beijing asylum into the Beijing Psychopathic Hospital, built a modern mental asylum in Nanjing, and supported the work already being done by medical missionaries in other cities. However, after the outbreak of war with Japan in 1937, most of the public and private psychopathic hospitals in China were forced into closure. By the time the Sino-Japanese War and subsequent civil war concluded, it was estimated that only 50 or 60 psychiatric practitioners remained in practice in mainland China. Modern Western psychiatric hospitals have introduced therapeutic and rehabilitative practices to China and significantly impacted the traditional Chinese psychiatric facilities that primarily functioned as confinement centers under police oversight. This shift has laid the groundwork for future advancements in China's psychiatric services.

醫療行動
與進步

隨著國民政府於 1937 年 11 月撤往重慶，抗日戰爭期間主要的醫療工作轉移至中國西南地區。美國政府及民間組織提供的青黴素生產技術、血庫及醫療物資，不僅拯救了無數中國人的生命，維持軍民的基本生存，也大大增強中國軍隊對抗日軍的力量。中國醫療人員的培訓，連同人道援助與聯合醫療行動，不僅促進中國醫療基礎設施的發展，也為現代醫療體系奠立基礎。

軍醫合作

1942 年秋天，許多國際醫療救護隊的醫生離開圖雲關，前往印度與緬甸，加入中國遠征軍 X 部隊。每個師包括三名軍官與兩名醫生。而留在中國的醫護人員則繼續跟隨林可勝博士在雲南前線服務，成為以昆明為基地的中國遠征軍 Y 部隊的一部分。

1943 年，中國紅十字會和中國軍隊在雲南部署了二十四支外科手術隊，其中包括來自公誼救護隊（Friends Ambulance Units）與英國紅十字會的三支外國醫療隊。在同盟國的指揮下，美軍、國際救援委員會（International Relief Committee）、中國紅十字會與國際醫療救護隊的醫生密切協作，統籌救援工作。1944 年 11 月，中國訓練與作戰指揮部（Chinese Training and Combat Command）正式成立，整合 Y 部隊與 Z 部隊的行動，藉此訓練並支援華中與華南地區的中國軍隊。

因為大多數技術精湛的醫生仍留在香港、上海和廣州等通商口岸，不願加入軍隊，合格的中國醫療人員極為稀缺。為了填補中國軍隊的醫療空缺，美國陸軍在中緬印戰區派遣受過專業訓練的醫療人員，並透過優先保全生命來強化軍事醫療服務。美軍中國戰區作戰司令部的一支醫療部隊與中國軍隊一同進入桂林，由美軍醫療人員提供高效的前線救治。該部隊擁有美國最先進的醫學知識與外科技術，不僅顯著提升了中國軍隊的醫療條件，也大大增強了士兵的士氣。有了即時的醫療援助，使中國士兵感到安心，進而在戰鬥中更加英勇無畏。

當全面抗戰爆發時，林可勝博士利用中國紅十字會爭取到國際援助與醫療支援，組織了第一批運往前線的醫療物資。隨後，他主持中國紅十字會醫療救護總隊的工作，總部設於貴州省的圖雲關，負責組建醫療隊伍、分發物資、並訓練應急人員。作為國民政府軍事委員會軍醫署署長，林博士在美國醫藥助華會的資助下，於1938年在圖雲關創立了戰時衛生人員訓練所。該單位的教職員都是他以前在協和醫學院的同事或教過的學生，負責訓練護理人員、擔架兵和前線衛生兵，為傷患提供即時救治。周美玉於1930年從協和醫學院護理系畢業，後來戰時衛生人員訓練所在貴陽成立時，護理科就是由她主持。 她與其他協和校友的努力，在這段動盪時期大幅提升了中國的軍事護理服務與教育水準。

戰時衛生人員訓練所與美國醫藥助華會合作，將中國軍醫體系中原本占主導地位的德式醫學模式調整為符合美國標準的體系，並在戰爭期間培訓了超過13,000名醫療人員，以滿足軍事與民間的醫療需求。該單位的衛生培訓計劃動員了當地助手參與公共衛生服務，並協助創辦多所女子護理學校及偏遠地區的衛生中心，成功在戰時維持了現代醫療體系的運作。此外，學校還組織了一支野戰救護營，該營配有軍醫與紅十字會人員，他們負責培訓當地志工，提升醫療物資與人員的協調能力，以此改善戰地醫療服務的運輸效率。

戰時中國的醫生短缺問題始終嚴峻。到1941年底，中國紅十字會救護總隊僅有181名醫生，其中包括部分來自國際醫療救護隊的外籍志願醫師。在延安，八路軍的百人規模白求恩國際和平醫院裡僅有九名醫生，而中國共產黨的新四軍則只有不到六十名合格醫師，卻要為超過九千萬人提供醫療服務。戰時衛生人員訓練所的畢業生加入陸軍衛生總隊與紅十字會救護總隊，前往前線與未被佔領地區服務。在這些地區，由戰地醫療急救學校培訓的護士與醫護人員承擔了大部分的醫療工作，成為戰時醫療體系的重要支柱。

輸血行動

戰時醫療中的輸血技術對外科手術、急救處理及特定疾病的治療至關重要。然而，尤其是在艱難的戰時環境中，穩定的供應輸血有賴血庫的建立。在美國醫藥助華會的支持下,兩名中國醫生前往哥倫比亞大學,師從約翰‧斯卡德(John Scudder)博士學習血漿製備技術,其中一人隨後在布林茅爾醫院(Bryn Mawr Hospital)進一步深造。此外,一位來自威斯康辛大學的華裔細菌學家也參與了該計畫。為支援中國的軍事現代化與戰爭,美國醫療助華會在美國募集了 817 名來自不同種族背景的捐血者,並將收集到的血液加工成血漿,運往中國。

在林可勝博士的努力與美國醫藥助華會的資助下,中國首座血庫於 1943 年在昆明成立,並配備了先進的技術來製備冷凍血漿。這一發展大幅增強了中國戰時的醫療救援能力。1944 年秋,雲南騰衝戰役戰況激烈,根據一名軍醫的報告,幾乎所有接受血漿輸注的傷兵都得以倖存,顯示了血庫對戰地救治的重大貢獻。

然而,挑戰隨之而來。傳統中國觀念視血液為身體不可或缺的一部分,認為失血會削弱元氣,甚至有違孝道,因而導致血庫難以募集血液,醫療用途的捐血亦極為罕見。尤其是士兵,他們普遍擔憂捐血會削弱自身體力。只有少數接受過西方醫學教育的城市精英能夠理解此一醫療概念並且捐血。

為了強調捐血在軍事醫療上的重要性,美國醫藥助華會與林可勝博士將這座機構命名為「陸軍軍醫署血庫」。儘管獲得中國軍方領導階層的支持,血液捐贈的推行仍面臨重重困難——士兵的抗拒心理、營養不良、惡劣的衛生環境及宣導不力,都使募血工作步履維艱。此外,電力與水源供應的不穩定,也嚴重影響了高壓滅菌器、離心機與冰箱等關鍵設備的運作。改用人力泵浦,並且將設備予以改裝,以燒炭提供動力,雖能勉強維持運作,但仍限制了血庫的處理能力。一次血漿污染事件更導致業務停滯數月,血庫不得不重新建立更嚴格的消毒程序與設備,以重建捐贈者的信心。

為了進一步提升低迷的捐血率,血庫的醫生、護士與流動捐血隊的助理親自前往軍營、學校與工地收集血液。這項行動顯著增加了捐血數量,到 1945 年戰爭結束時,流動捐血隊募集的血液已佔總量的 92%。此外,血庫還發起宣傳運動,喚起民眾的利他精神與愛國情懷,並以簡單的食物作為獎勵，鼓勵更多人參與。來自西南聯合大學的學生及電力、鐵路公司工人踴躍響應，為戰時中國提供了寶貴的民間血液捐贈。

戰場上的外科手術

　　中緬印戰區完全依賴穿越喜馬拉雅山脈的空運（即「駝峰航線」）來維持後勤補給。瘧疾迅速蔓延，但藥物極為短缺。戰場橫跨山地、叢林與河谷，再加上季風帶來的暴雨，造成地面運輸幾乎無法運作。由於X光機與顯微鏡等醫療設備無法在敵軍炮火範圍內運送，這些器材只能由士兵背負、馱獸載運，或透過空投抵達戰場。因此，戰場手術大多在便攜式外科單位或臨時搭建的醫院內進行，這些醫療站通常設於帳篷或徵用建築內，以便在前線附近提供即時的外科處置。在華東戰區，僅有四個可移動外科醫院，每個單位配有兩名外科醫生與十八名醫務兵。醫務兵負責為傷者解開衣物、清理傷口、進行初步清創，並在必要時施打靜脈麻醉。外科醫生則在病床間迅速來回，縫合淺表傷口、摘除眼球，或根據需求進行手臂或腿部截肢手術。

　　1945年5月，美國陸軍中國戰區作戰司令部的軍醫班傑明・伯克上校（Colonel Benjamin J. Birk）與其他顧問一同前往桂林淪陷後成為最前線戰鬥基地的芷江，以及中國戰區作戰司令部東線司令部所在地安江。他們視察了中美陸軍醫院，肯定醫療團隊在巨大壓力下所完成的高水準外科手術，以及在面對大量等待手術傷患時，仍能維持良好醫療服務的表現。

接種疫苗

　　為了應對華北的地方性鼠疫疫情，北洋政府於1919年成立了中央防疫處，透過製造疫苗與血清來壓制鼠疫。後來對日抗戰於1937年全面爆發，藥品與醫療物資的短缺、醫療基礎設施與衛生條件的缺乏、惡劣的生活環境、營養不良，以及戰時大量軍人與難民的遷徙，導致霍亂在擁擠的城市與難民營中爆發，瘧疾與細菌性痢疾則在中國部隊中迅速蔓延。

在此情況下，疫苗接種仍是國家衛生行政機構的首要任務。

到了國民政府時代，中央防疫處得以進口標準疫苗樣本與設備，並在昆明、貴陽與蘭州重建生化實驗室，實在是有賴各國組織援助，例如丹麥國家血清研究所（State Serum Institute）、美國國家衛生研究院（National Institutes of Health）、英國醫學研究委員會（Medical Research Council），而國際聯盟（League of Nations）的幫助尤為重要。1937年至1945年間，中央防疫處利用實驗動物製造了數百萬劑天花、霍亂、傷寒等疾病的疫苗。同時，中國紅十字會也在貴陽建立了自己的疫苗製造設施，至1943年已能每年生產六百萬劑疫苗，涵蓋霍亂、傷寒、白喉、破傷風與斑疹傷寒等疾病。

1941年，國民政府對外宣傳免疫接種是對抗日軍可能發動生物戰的重要武器，並強制前線軍人與後方民眾接種霍亂、痢疾與傷寒的預防疫苗。儘管疫苗接種確實降低了疫情的嚴重程度與發生頻率，但戰時的大規模接種工作仍面臨諸多困難，包括日軍空襲、運輸延誤、疫苗污染與過期、衛生設施不足，以及民眾對疫苗接種的抗拒等問題。

盤尼西林

昆明是美國陸軍航空隊在中國的空運中心，地理位置上的優勢使得中央防疫處的工作人員能夠接觸到如《柳葉刀》（*The Lancet*）等最新的國外醫學期刊，並得知西方已成功研發出療效豐碩的盤尼西林。1944年春，在洛克斐勒基金會的支持下，兩名中央防疫處人員前往印度考察當地的公共衛生機構，返國時帶回來十株來自英美的盤尼西林菌株。同時，一位從美國威斯康辛大學返國的中國微生物學家又帶回三株菌種。中央防疫處還從美國伊利諾州皮奧里亞（Peoria）的北部地區研究實驗室（Northern Regional Research Laboratory）取得了盤尼西林菌株，該實驗室當時正致力於研發其發酵培養技術。中央防疫處的工作人員隨即展開了培養與提煉盤尼西林菌株的研究工作。

美國醫藥助華會、國民政府衛生署與中國紅十字會合作，撥款從美國購買醫療物資與設備。由於無法直接購買盤尼西林運往中國，美國醫藥助華會與美國援華工業合作社委員會（Indusco）在紐約共同設立了一座小型工廠，不僅試圖為中國提供盤尼西林的製造方法，更希望將抗生素的研究與生產技術引入中國本土。

這間工廠在資源極度匱乏的中國戰時條件下，利用僅有的材料與設備，研發出粗製與精製青黴素的生產方法。工廠還訓練了一位在約翰霍普金斯大學取得博士學位的中國細菌學家，教授其青黴素生產技術。該學者返國後，負責培訓人員，並在中國未淪陷地區建立新的生產實驗室。

然而，由於技術上的困難，國民政府的中央防疫處未能自行成功製造青黴素。為解決問題，美國醫藥助華會邀請美國細菌學家前來討論在中國戰時環境中培養青黴素所面臨的技術瓶頸，並確認青黴素培養基中的關鍵成分——「玉米浸出液」在中國境內無法取得。經過美國醫藥助華會提供約一千九百萬元法幣的資助，以及多次實驗嘗試替代品之後，中央防疫處終於在1944年9月成功生產出五瓶青黴素，每瓶含有五千個牛津單位。此外，根據《租借法案》的安排，美國陸軍航空隊於1944年8月運送了465瓶青黴素（總計4650萬單位）至中國給各家醫院。至此，青黴素與磺胺類藥物從1944年開始終於在中國戰場上得以用於治療感染，極大改善了前線傷患的救治情況。

口腔保健

北京協和醫學院在戰時中國維持了牙科部門，對於牙科專業人員的培訓與現代牙科技術的推廣可說是貢獻良多。抗日戰爭全面爆發後，中國的牙科醫療體系幾乎被摧毀。部分國際牙醫，如俄籍牙醫迪米崔·阿方斯基（Dimitri Afonsky），以及駐華美國陸軍牙科部隊，協助為中國軍人提供牙科治療、牙外科服務及相關教育。美國陸軍牙科部隊除了為美軍與盟軍提供牙科服務，也逐步擴展至中國戰區（原屬中緬印戰區）。作為中國戰區的牙科軍官，理查·達比中校（Lieutenant Colonel Richard D. Darby）負責全區的牙科服務工作。他的職責包括跨越險峻的「駝峰航線」從印度向中國運輸牙科醫療物資，以應對中國戰區幅員遼闊、補給困難的挑戰。

醫療部門所配備的器械、儀器與物資，主要用於野戰醫院中一般性的牙科手術與治療。儘管設備與物資極為短缺，1944年初仍設立了一座牙科修復實驗室。由於缺乏現成設備，實驗室不得不自行建造乙炔發生器，以確保氣體供應；直到1944年末，才成功安裝了電石氣系統。該實驗室僅有兩名牙科軍官與七名士兵，卻肩負起製作全口與局部義齒、修補假牙、製作牙橋等任務，以滿足中國軍人的牙科需求。此外，行動牙科診所也在帳篷或臨時改建的建築內搭建完成，使牙科團隊能接近前線地區，提供拔牙、補牙與緊急處置等基本但至關重要的牙科服務。

有鑑於中國軍隊普遍缺乏牙科照護，美國陸軍牙科部隊的軍官率先為中國軍醫及藥劑軍官開設第一個牙科訓練課程。第一期課程於1943年11月在雲南大理舉行，為期一個月，內容專注於口腔外科基礎與口腔疾病治療。考量部分學員需長途跋涉，甚至花費二十天才能抵達大理，美國陸軍牙科部隊講師亦主動前往各個國軍部隊的派駐地，開設精簡課程，使中國部隊具備基本的牙科醫療能力。

1944年4月，美國陸軍牙科部隊在中國桂林設立了另一所牙科訓練學校，學生人數限定為十二人。參訓者中包含兩名中國軍隊的女性護理軍官，分別為少尉與中尉軍階。至1944年7月25日因日軍猛烈攻勢而被迫停辦前，共有兩期、二十四名學員順利結業，另有十二名學員僅接受了部分訓練。

精神醫療支援

除了貧困、疾病、天災與戰爭所帶來的巨大破壞，戰爭還對倖存的中國人造成深遠的心理創傷。儘管戰時中國極需精神醫療支援，但實際上的資源卻相當有限，這不僅是因為醫療資源主要集中於身體健康，也受到社會對心理疾病的污名化與專業人員缺乏等因素影響。在19世紀末至20世紀初，西方來華的醫療傳教士與醫師是最早將現代精神醫學引入中國的群體之一。1898年，美國醫療傳教士暨慈善家嘉約翰（John G.

Kerr）協助創建了中國第一所現代精神疾病治療機構，名為惠愛醫癲院（Canton Hospital for the Insane），設立於廣州。來自奧地利的神經精神科醫師韓芬（Fanny Halpern）則與上海當地精英合作，創辦了普慈療養院（Shanghai Mercy Hospital），成為上海第一所精神病醫院。

受到美國模式影響，國民政府將原有的北平收容所改建為北平市立精神病療養院，並於南京興建一所現代化精神病療養院，同時也支持其他城市由醫療傳教士所推動的精神醫療事業。然而，自 1937 年抗日戰爭爆發後，多數公私立精神病院被迫關閉。至抗戰及隨後的國共內戰結束時，據估計，中國大陸僅剩五、六十位精神科醫師仍在執業。現代西方精神病院所引入的治療與復健制度，對中國傳統以監禁與警察管理為主的精神病收容體系產生了深遠影響，也為中國未來心理醫療服務的發展奠定了基礎。

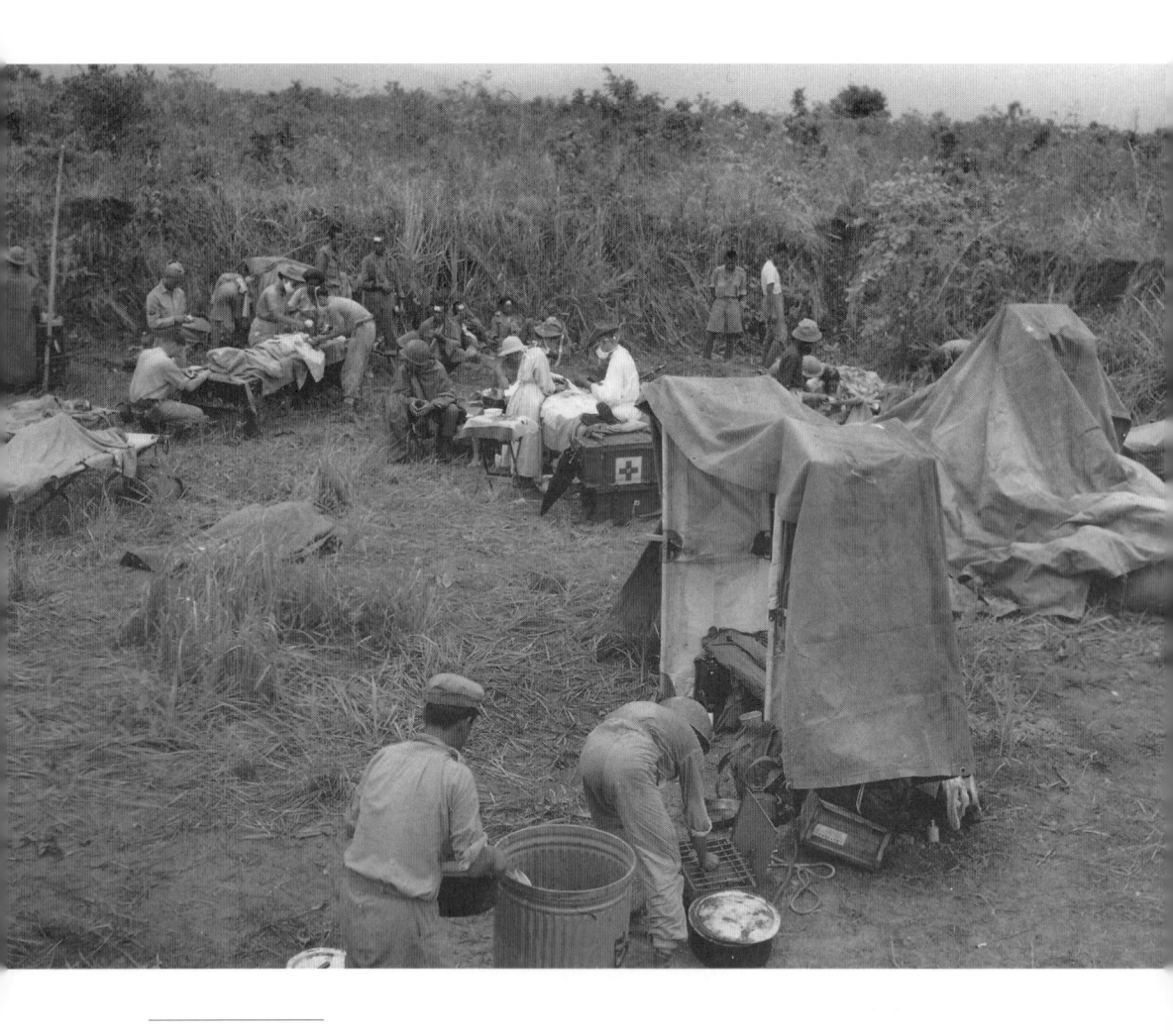

Medical personnel of the Seagraves Hospital Unit were preparing for the surgical operations in a field near the Mytikyina Airfield, Burma.

緬甸密支那機場附近的原野上,海格雷夫斯醫療部隊的醫療人員正在進行手術的準備工作。

Date of Photo 時間:May 19, 1944
Credits 來源:美國國家檔案館 Photo Courtesy of National Archives

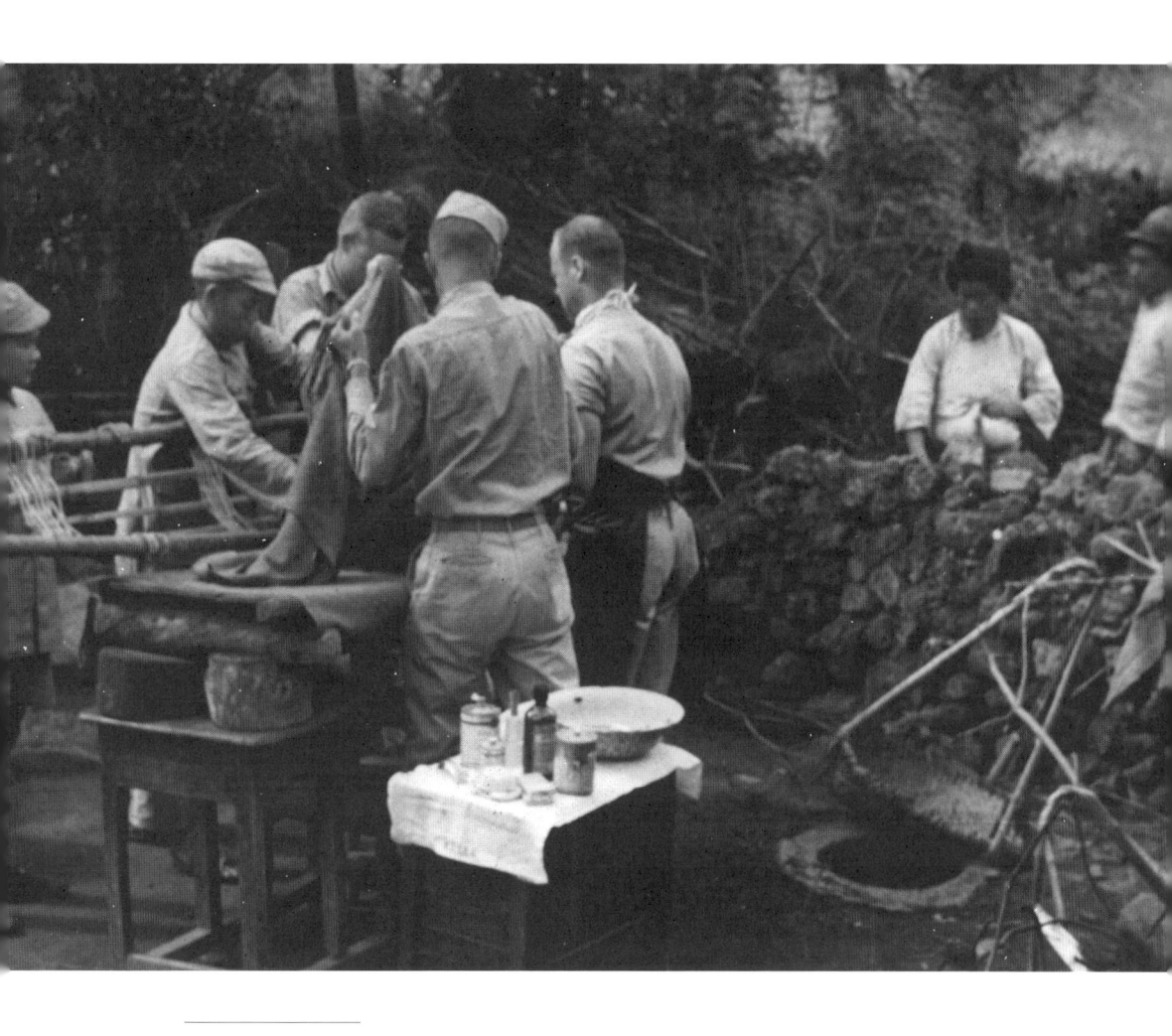

A United States Army surgeon had just finished surgery on a wounded Chinese soldier at a makeshift operating table in a Chinese farmyard. The patient was being lifted to a stretcher.

一位美國陸軍外科醫生,在中國農場的臨時手術台上剛為一名受傷的中國士兵完成手術。病人正被抬到擔架上。

Date of Photo 時間:September 18, 1944
Credits 來源:美國國家檔案館 Photo Courtesy of National Archives

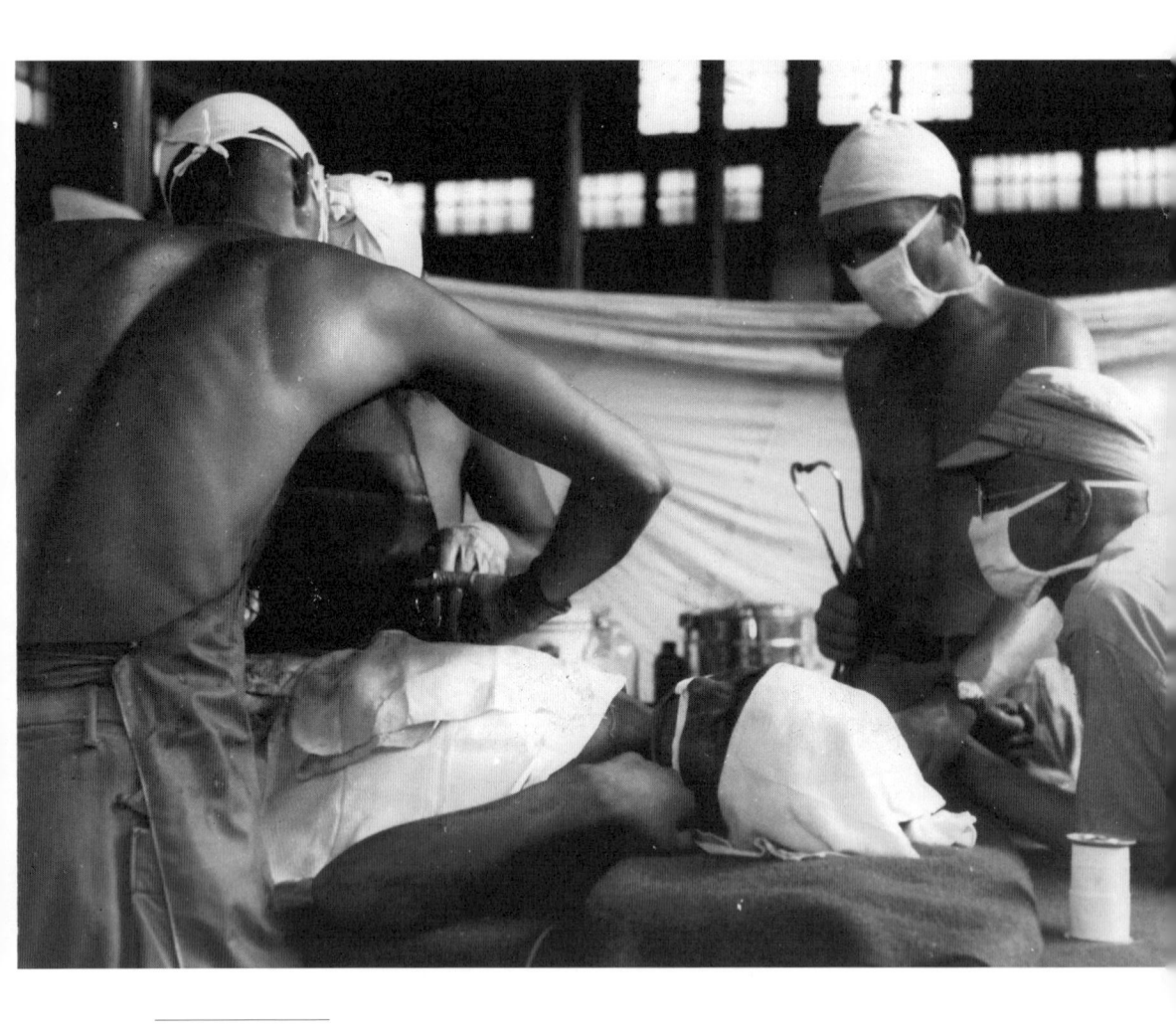

A wounded Chinese soldier was undergoing a surgery in an American-portable surgical hospital in the recaptured city of Guilin.

一名受傷的中國士兵正在美國提供的移動式手術醫院中接受手術,該醫院位於國軍收復的桂林市。

Date of Photo 時間:August 1, 1945
Credits 來源:美國國家檔案館 Photo Courtesy of National Archives

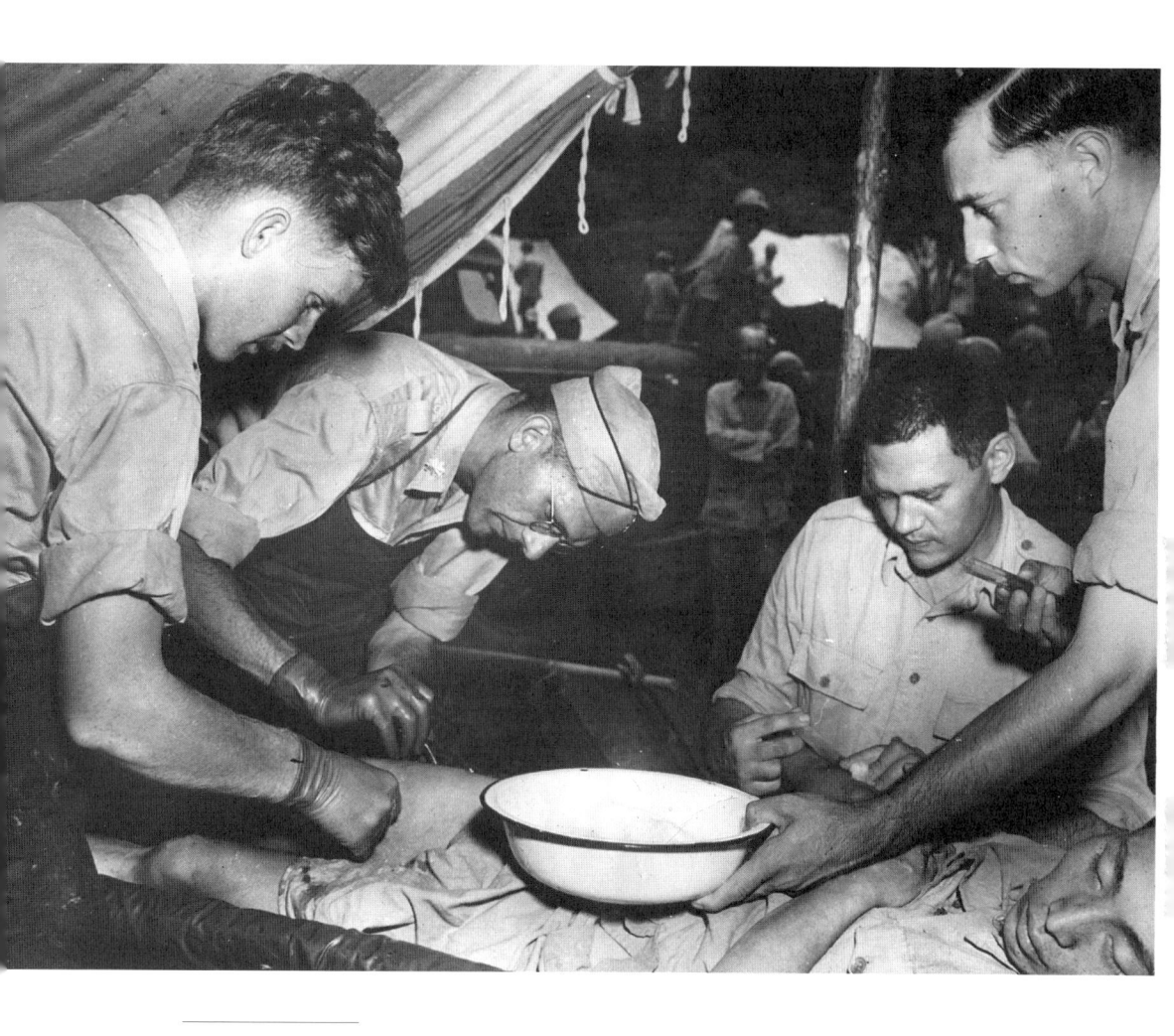

An American surgeon, assisted by three United States Army medical corpsmen, was removing shrapnel from the leg of a Chinese soldier wounded in the Battle of Songshan, Yunnan, at an emergency dressing station.

在急救包紮站裡,一位美國外科醫生在三名美軍醫療兵的協助下,正為一名於雲南松山戰役中受傷的中國士兵取出腿上的彈片。

Date of Photo 時間:October 2, 1944
Credits 來源:美國國家檔案館 Photo Courtesy of National Archives

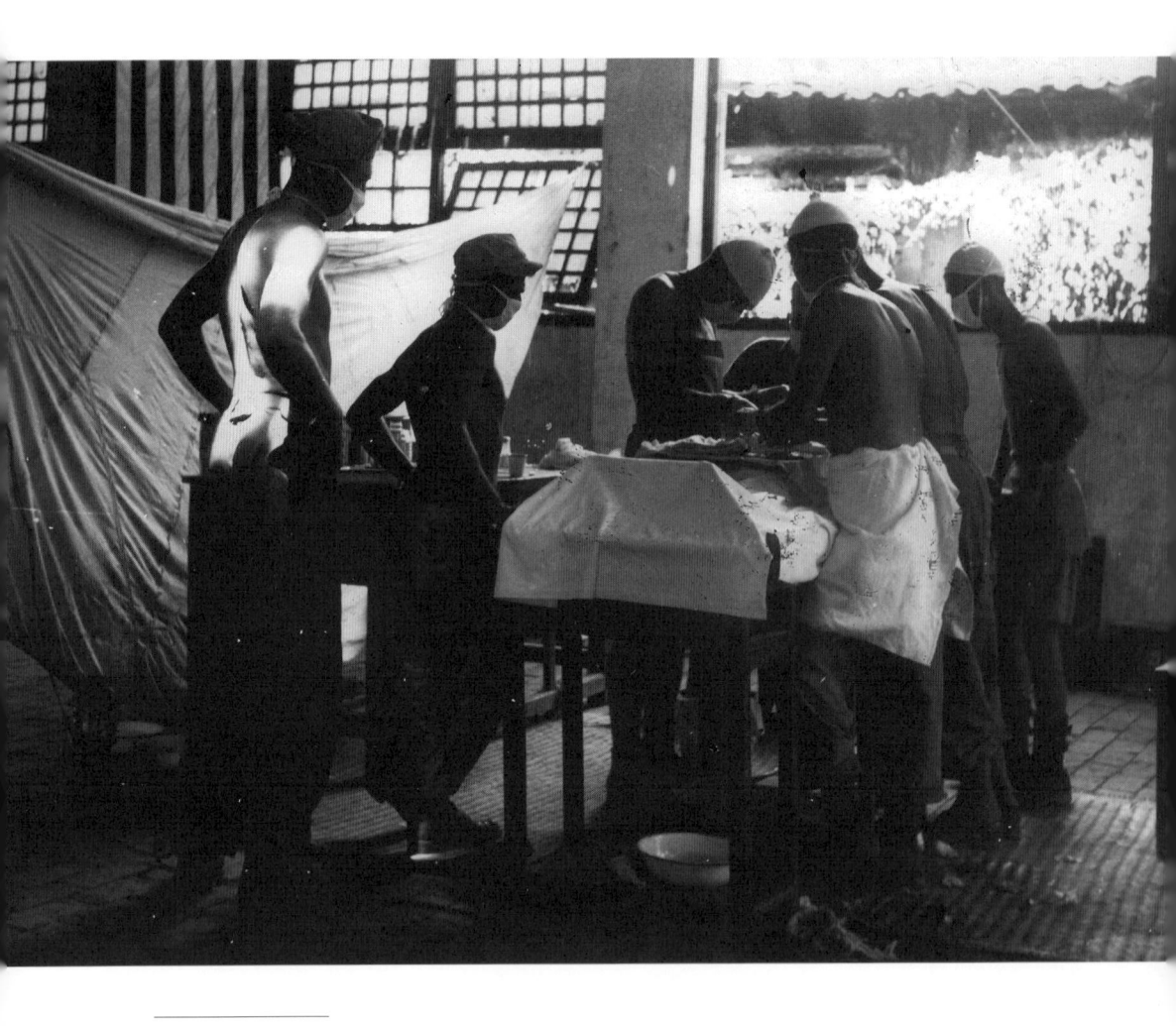

A United States Army surgeon had just finished surgery on a wounded Chinese soldier at a makeshift operating table in a Chinese farmyard.

一位美國陸軍外科醫生在中國農場裡的臨時手術台上,剛為一名受傷的中國士兵完成手術。

Date of Photo 時間:不詳 N/A
Credits 來源:美國國家檔案館 Photo Courtesy of National Archives

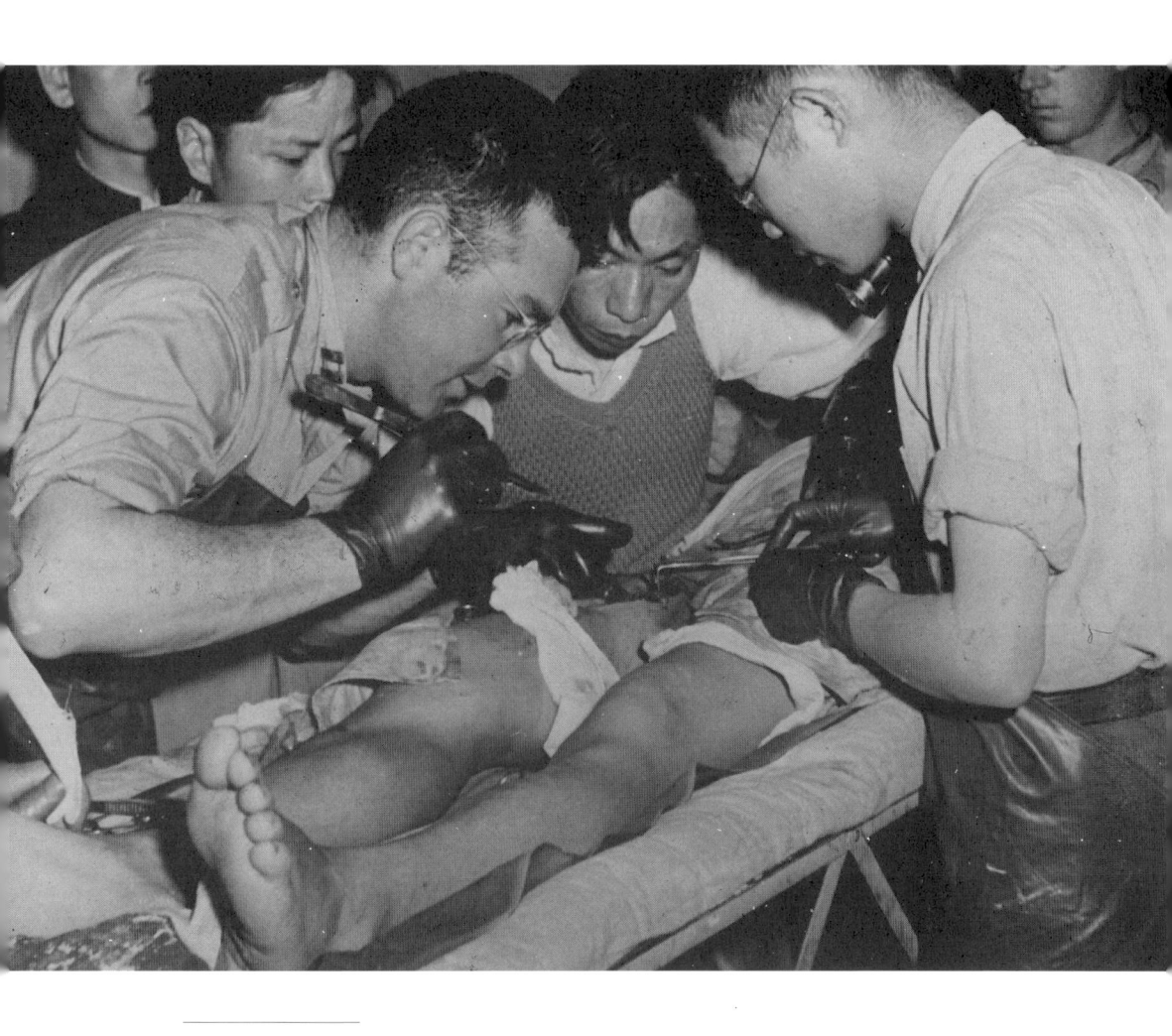

A United States Army surgeon was operating on the leg of a Chinese soldier wounded by Japanese shells during Chinese defense of the United States airfield at Zijiang, Hunan.

一名中國士兵防守位於湖南芷江的美國空軍基地時,被日軍炮彈擊中腿部,一名美國陸軍外科醫生正在為其進行手術。

Date of Photo 時間:June 24, 1945
Credits 來源:美國國家檔案館 Photo Courtesy of National Archives

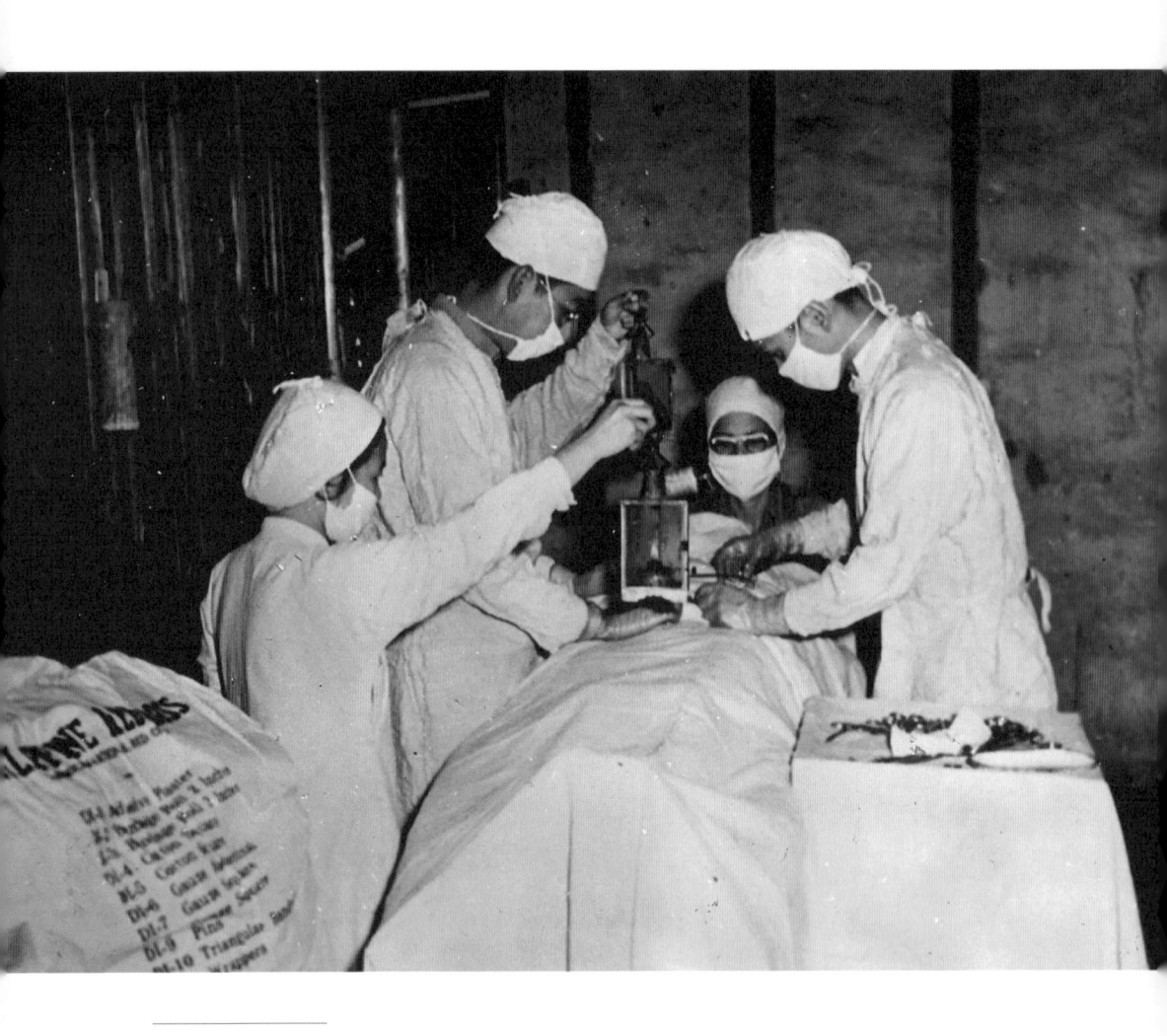

Two Chinese doctors were conducting an emergency operation by the light of an oil lamp held by a young nurse.

兩名中國醫生正在進行緊急手術，旁邊有個年輕護理人員手持油燈為其照明。

Date of Photo 時間：不詳 N/A
Credits 來源：美國國家檔案館 Photo Courtesy of National Archives

At the Chinese Training Center, American medical personnel were administering an anti-tetanus shot to a Chinese soldier with a bandaged head injury.

在中國訓練中心，美國醫療人員正在為一名頭部受傷且已完成包紮的中國士兵施打破傷風疫苗。

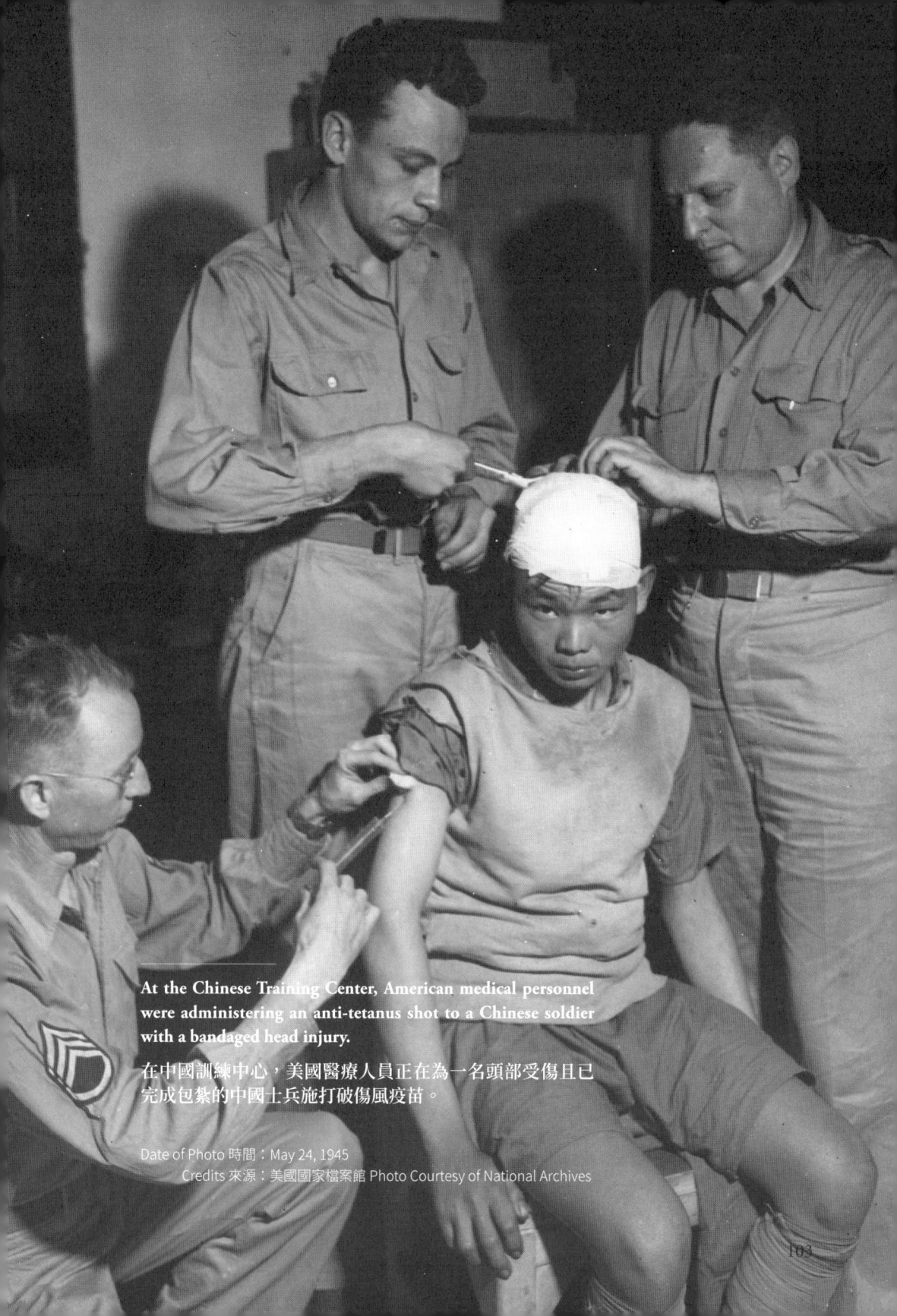

Date of Photo 時間：May 24, 1945
Credits 來源：美國國家檔案館 Photo Courtesy of National Archives

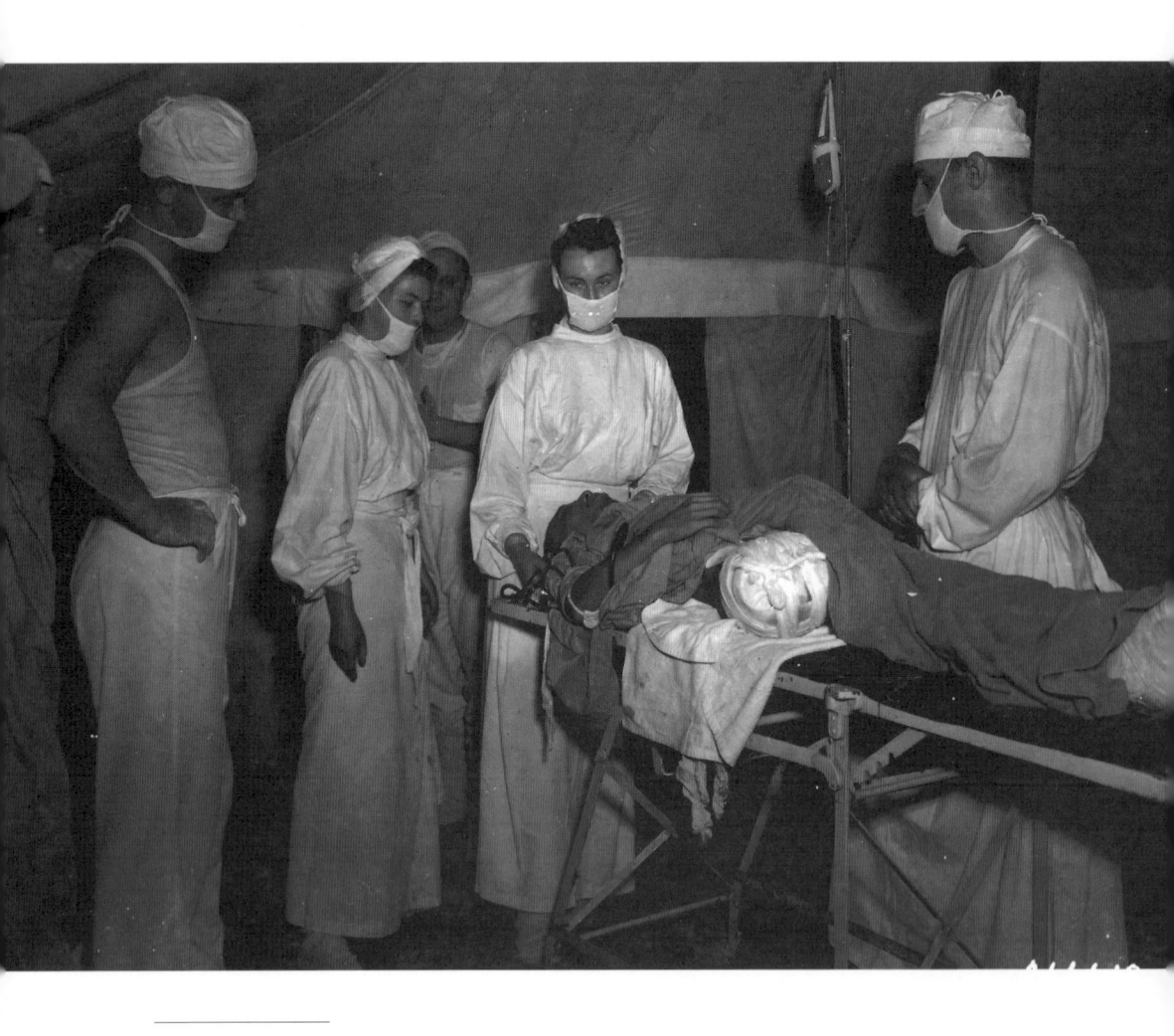

This wounded Chinese soldier was receiving blood plasma after having his right leg amputated. He was injured while fighting Japanese force in Mogaung Valley, Burma.

一名中國士兵在緬甸孟拱河谷與日本軍隊作戰時受傷,其右腿被截肢後正在接受輸血。

Date of Photo 時間:May 23, 1944
Credits 來源:美國國家檔案館 Photo Courtesy of National Archives

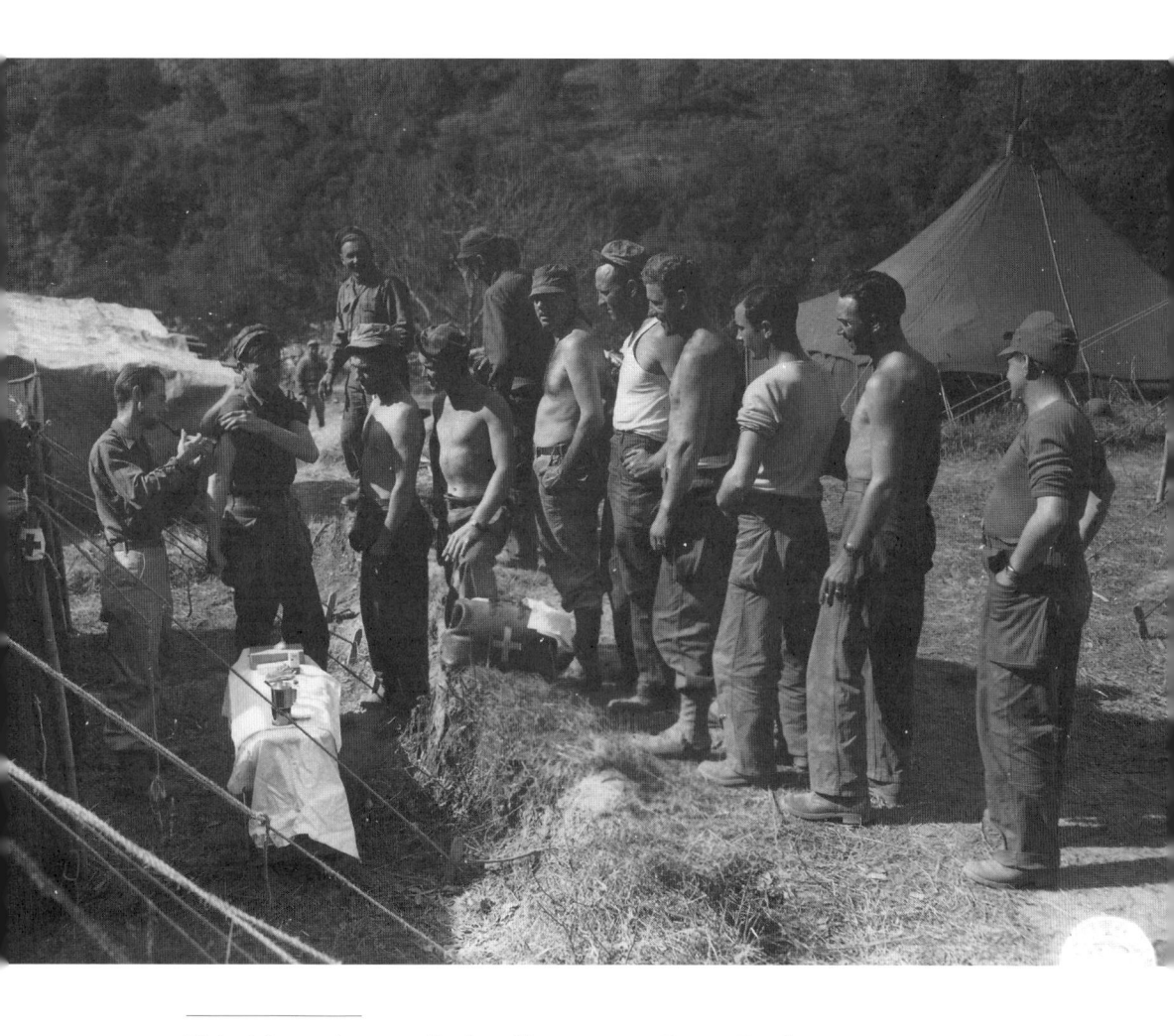

United States Army medical staff were giving Burma Road engineers vaccine shots to protect them against tropical diseases. They were building a new land supply route for the vital war materiel to be shipped from India's supply depots to China's fighting forces.

美國陸軍醫療人員正在為參與修建滇緬公路的工程師注射熱帶疾病疫苗。這條新建的陸路補給線旨在將戰爭物資從印度運送至中國前線。

Date of Photo 時間：不詳 N/A
Credits 來源：美國國家檔案館 Photo Courtesy of National Archives

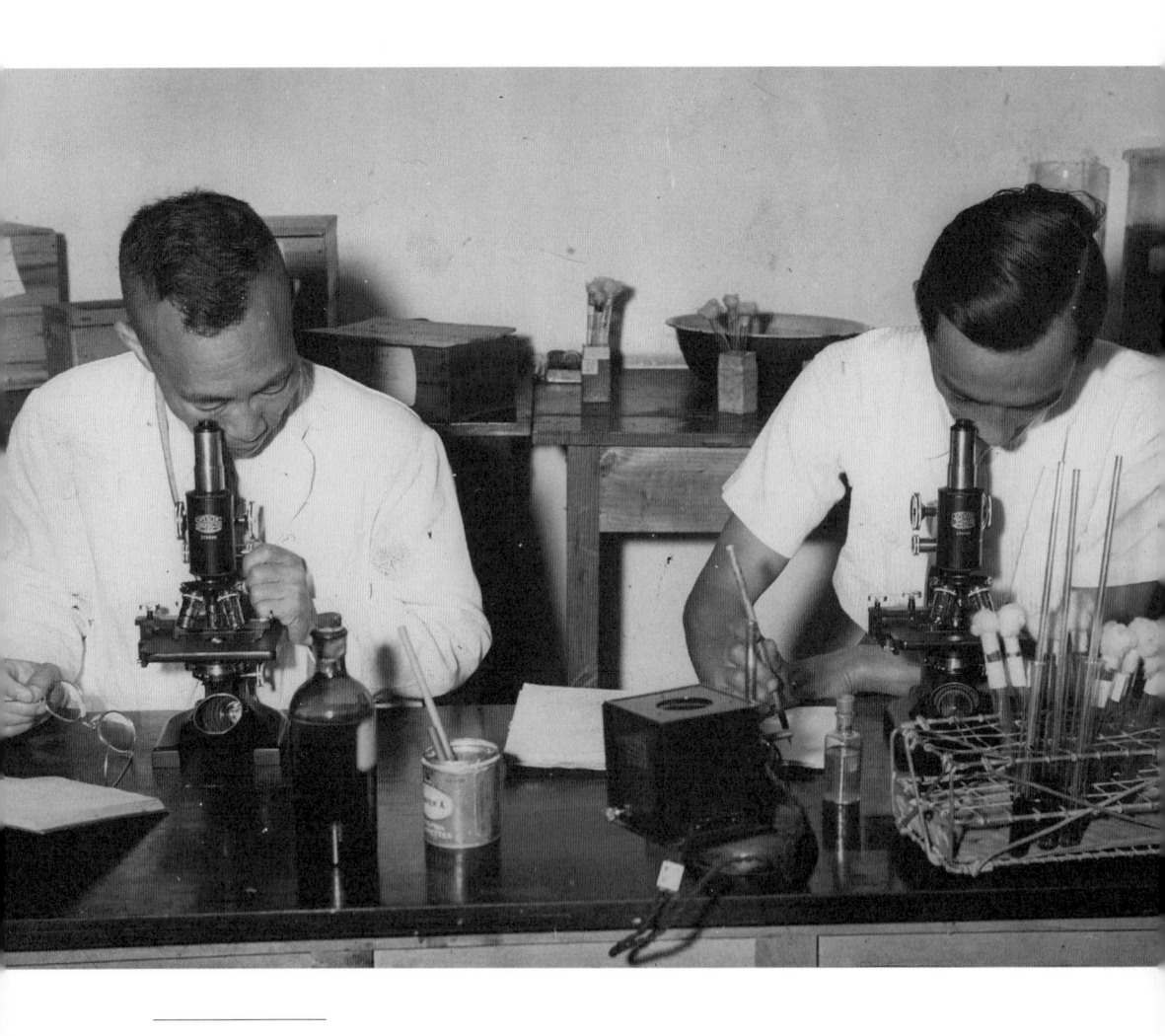

In a Chinese hospital, two Chinese doctors were conducting research on vaccines and serums using the modern microscopes that the American Red Cross sent to the Chinese Red Cross.

在一家中國醫院內,兩位中國醫生正使用由美國紅十字會贈予中國紅十字會的現代顯微鏡,進行疫苗與血清方面的研究。

Date of Photo 時間:不詳 N/A
Credits 來源:美國國家檔案館 Photo Courtesy of National Archives

Two Catholic nuns were wrapping the bandages of a wounded Chinese soldier's head, who was injured in the Battle of Taierzhuang, Shangdong and praying for him.

兩名天主教修女正在為一名在台兒莊戰役中受傷的中國士兵包紮頭部，同時為他祈禱。

Date of Photo 時間：May 24, 1938
Credits 來源：美國國家檔案館 Photo Courtesy of National Archives

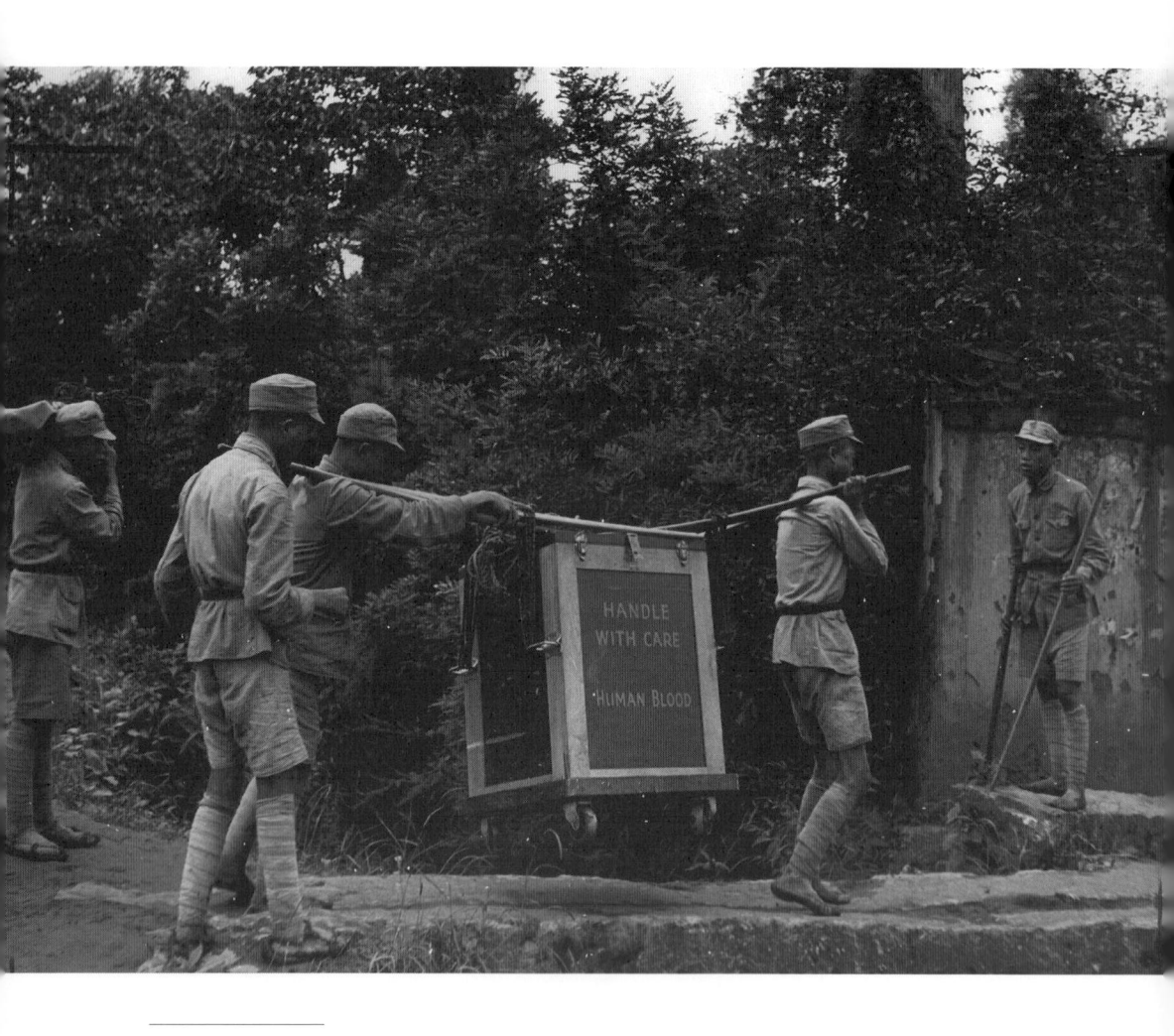

Chinese soldiers were carrying a heavy bottle-filled refrigerator to a Chinese Army headquarter where Chinese troops donate their blood to save the lives of their comrades at the various fronts.

中國士兵正將一個裝滿瓶子的冰箱抬往中國軍隊總部，讓部隊士兵得以在各個前線踴躍捐血，以挽救戰友的生命。

Date of Photo 時間：不詳 N/A
Credits 來源：美國國家檔案館 Photo Courtesy of National Archives

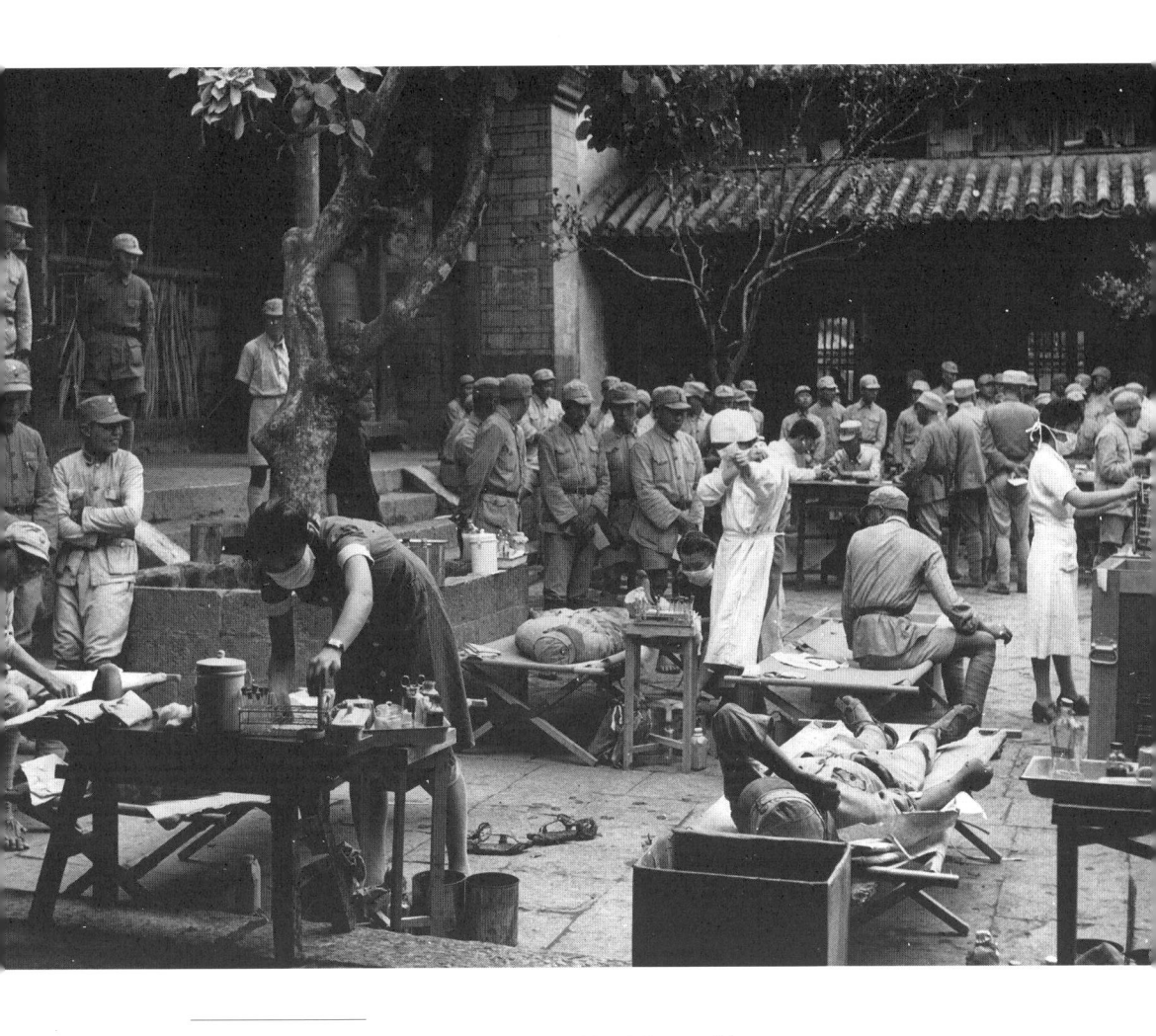

Chinese doctors and nurses were taking blood from soldiers in the courtyard of an old Chinese temple serving as the ward.

在一座改建為病房的古老寺廟院落中,中國醫生與護理人員正為士兵抽血。

Date of Photo 時間:不詳 N/A
Credits 來源:美國國家檔案館 Photo Courtesy of National Archives

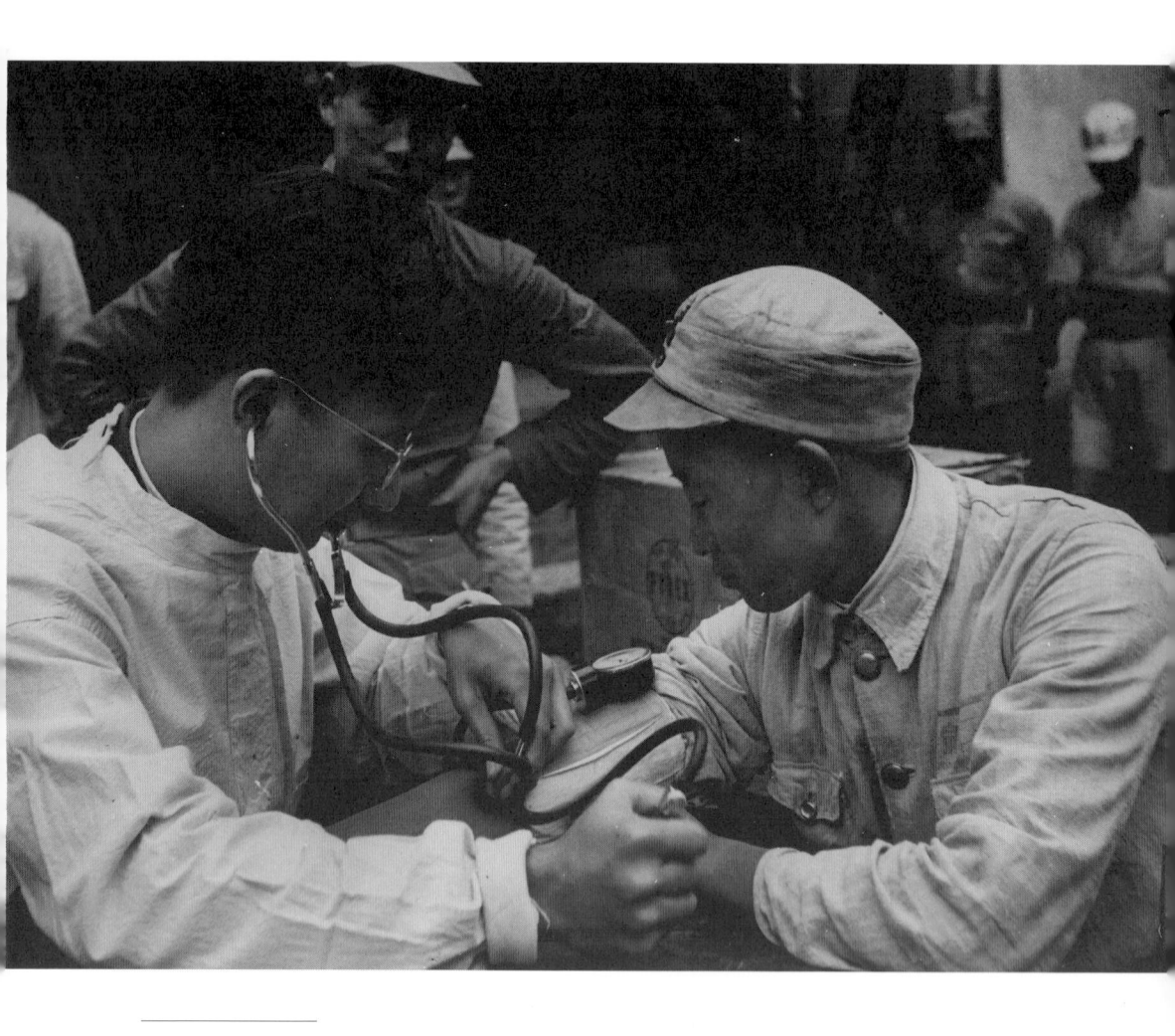

Chinese doctors and nurses were giving the hemoglobin and blood pressure test to a Chinese soldier before taking his blood.

在為一名中國士兵抽血前,中國醫生與護士正為他進行血紅素與血壓檢測。

Date of Photo 時間:不詳 N/A
Credits 來源:美國國家檔案館 Photo Courtesy of National Archives

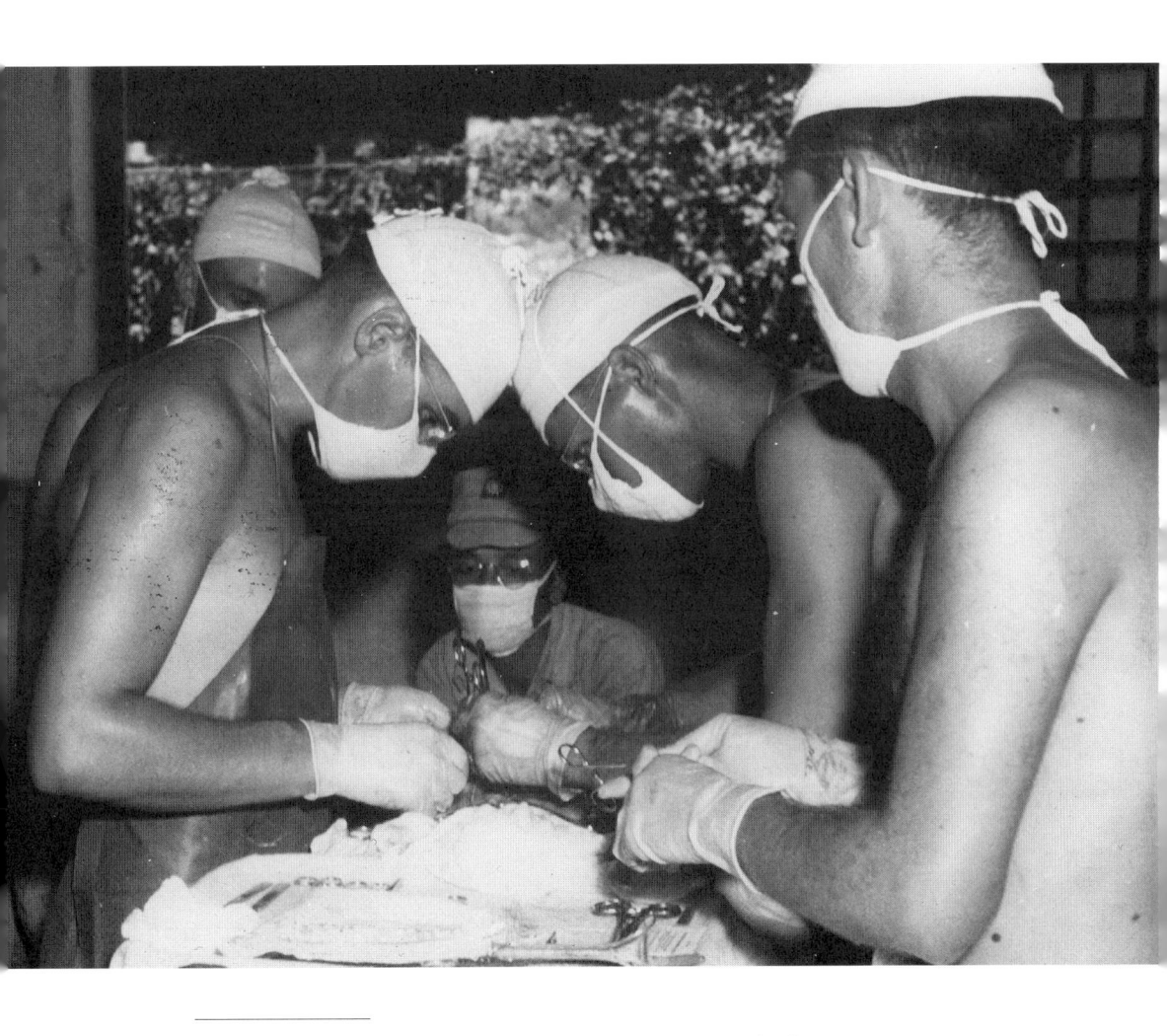

An American surgeon and corpsmen from the American Medical Unit were operating on a Chinese soldier in a portable hospital set up in the reoccupied city of Guilin.

在國軍重新收復的桂林市內一座移動式醫院中,一名美國外科醫生與數名美國陸軍醫務兵正在為一位中國士兵進行手術。

Date of Photo 時間:August 21, 1945
Credits 來源:美國國家檔案館 Photo Courtesy of National Archives

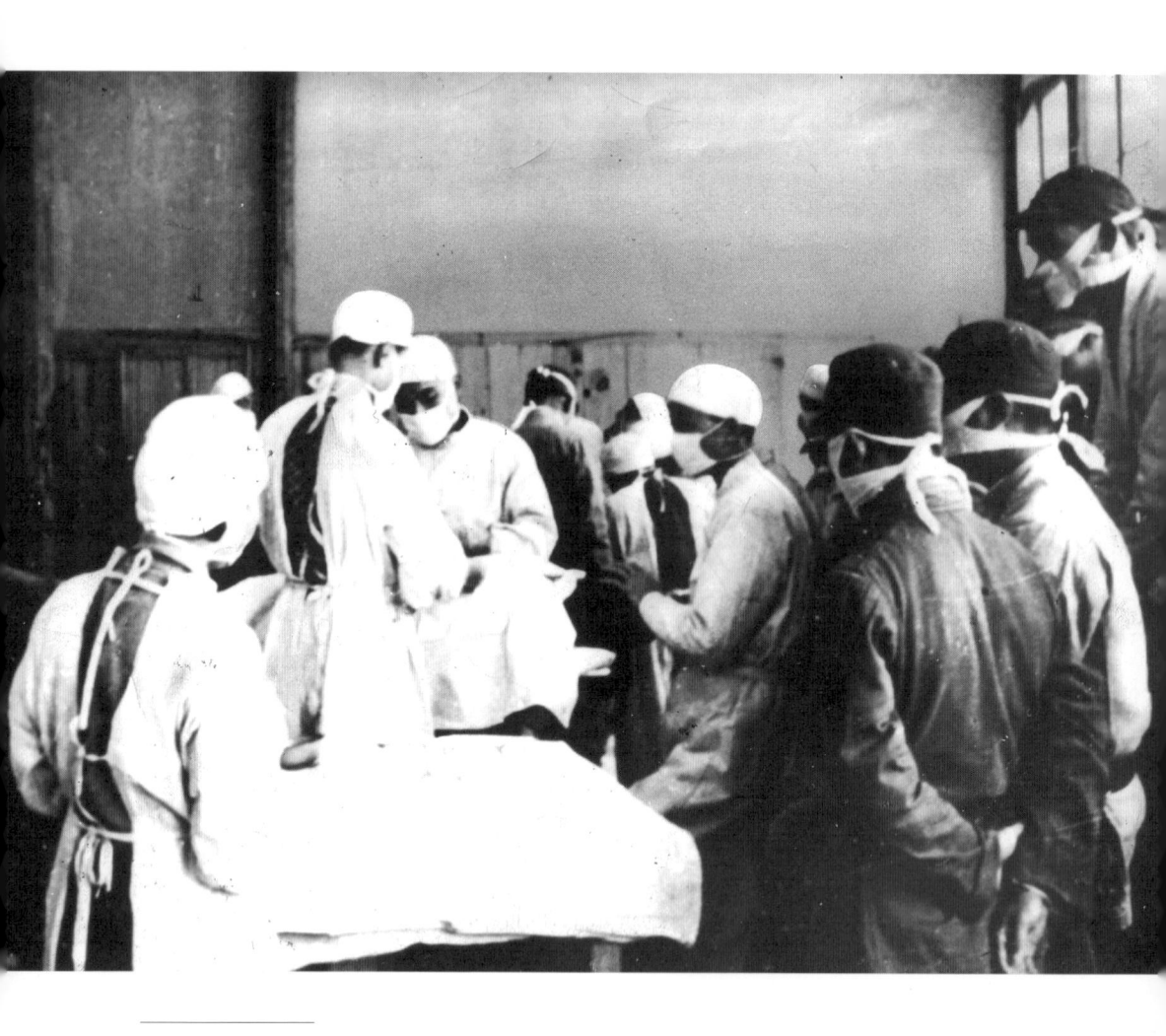

Chinese doctors and interns worked tirelessly at an emergency Chinese hospital behind the front lines.

在前線後方的緊急醫院裡，中國醫生與實習醫生們正日以繼夜地進行傷員搶救工作。

Date of Photo 時間：不詳 N/A
Credits 來源：美國國家檔案館 Photo Courtesy of National Archives

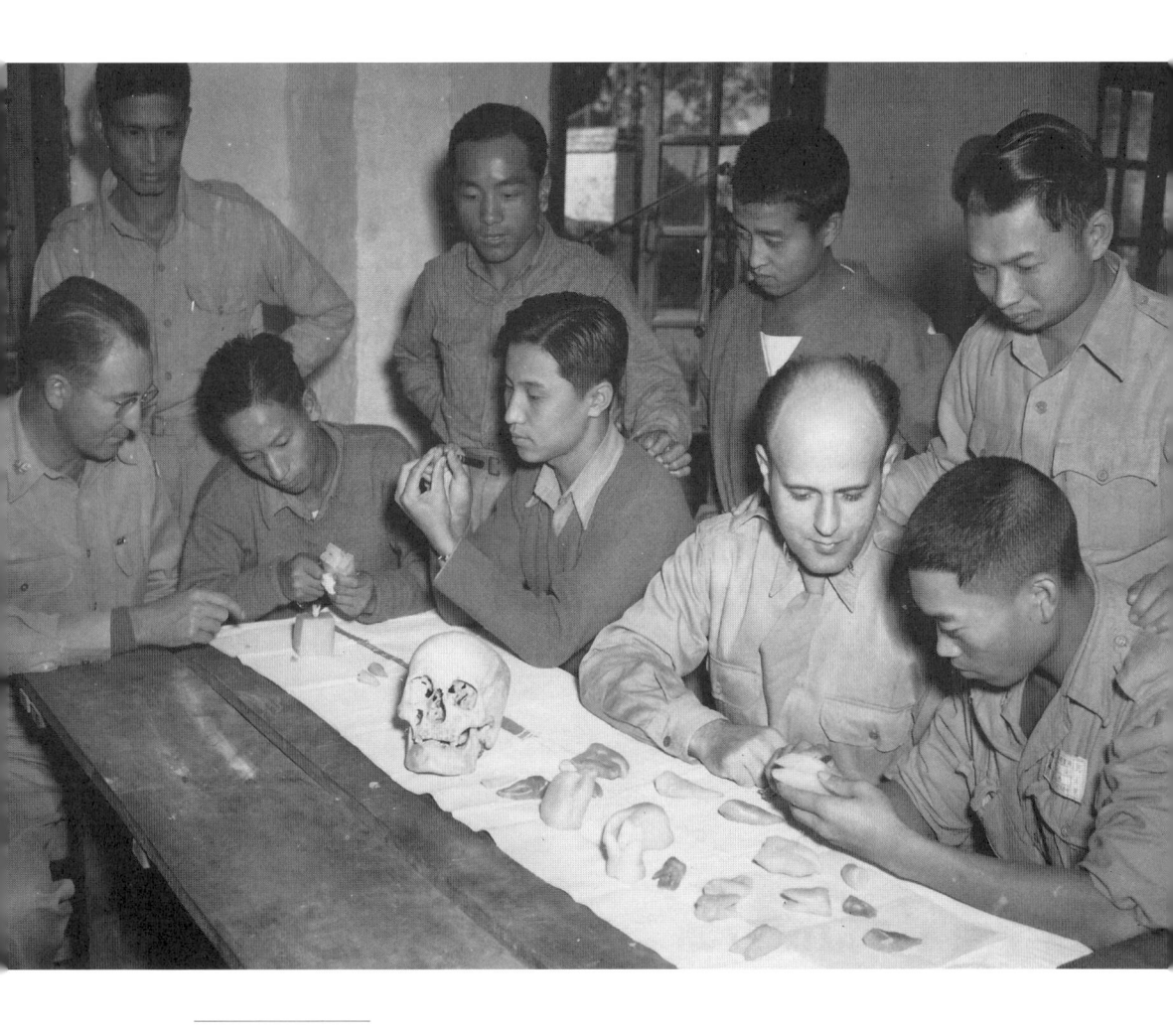

Future Chinese dental officers were getting thorough dental course training in New York. They were carving soap models of different types of teeth.

幾位即將成為牙科軍醫的中國人,正在紐約接受完整的牙科訓練課程。他們用肥皂雕刻各種齒模,以練習牙齒結構與修復技術。

Date of Photo 時間:November 28,1944
Credits 來源:美國國家檔案館 Photo Courtesy of National Archives

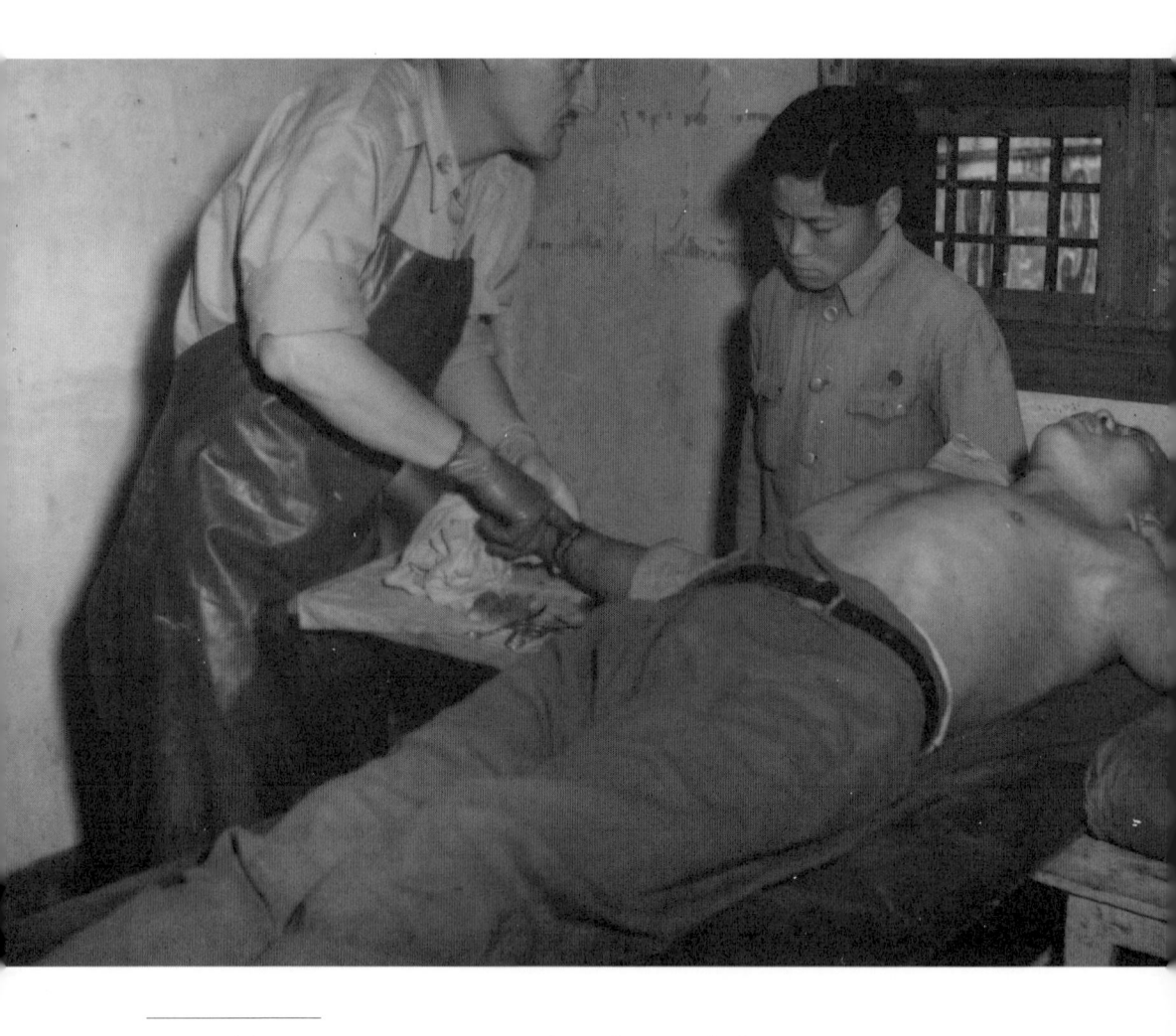

A United States Army surgeon was probing the wound of a Chinese soldier using his fingers.

一名美國陸軍外科醫生正在用手指探查一名中國士兵的傷口。

Date of Photo 時間：不詳 N/A
Credits 來源：美國國家檔案館 Photo Courtesy of National Archives

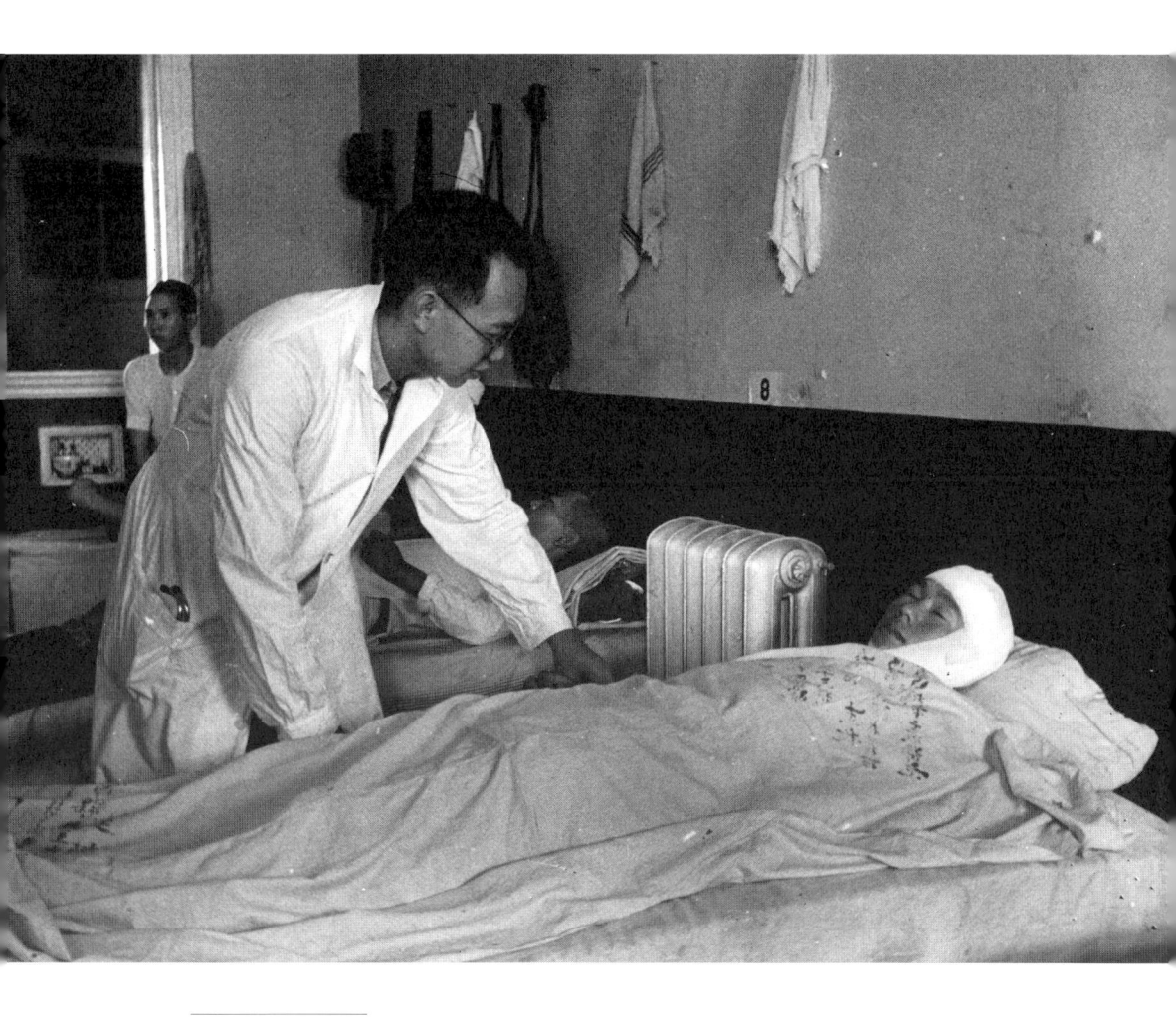

A Chinese soldier was recovering in the hospital under the careful attention of a Chinese doctor.

一名中國士兵於醫院中接受治療,在一名中國醫生的細心照料下逐漸康復。

Date of Photo 時間:不詳 N/A
Credits 來源:美國國家檔案館 Photo Courtesy of National Archives

WORKING AND LIVING CONDITIONS

Malnutrition

During World War II, China was, compared to the west, a relatively impoverished agrarian economy that struggled to meet the basic dietary needs of its more than 500 million citizens. The dire nutritional status of the Chinese was exacerbated by a strict embargo for imported relief goods, the destruction unleashed by modern warfare, and devastating droughts. Widespread malnutrition and starvation became core challenges that confounded the delivery of basic medical care.

Several physicians of the International Medical Relief Corps (IMRC) documented the security of malnutrition in wartime China. In a 1939 report from Chinese Medical Relief Corps Unit 32, Dr. Erich Mamlok mentioned: "Due to the chronic malnutrition affecting most of the patients, medical work became much more difficult. Autopsies conducted by Dr. Wu with special permission from the military authorities revealed signs of chronic malnutrition in nearly every case, including the disappearance of subcutaneous fat and omental fat, anemia, intestinal atrophy, soft bones, and so on. In some cases of enteritis, the inflammation of the intestine was so mild that the patients must have died of malnutrition rather than as a result of enteritis. This deficiency is a lack of essential nutrients, particularly albumin and vitamins."

The Chinese Red Cross estimated that the daily diet provided by the Guomindang Nationalist Party to the Chinese Army included 953 grams of rice, 273 grams of vegetables, ten grams of lard and thirteen grams of salt. From a practical standpoint, this meant that the soldiers were trying to survive on two meals a day consisting of a dish of vegetables with some meat or, more commonly, just soup, rice, and rice-water porridge. Furthermore, the corruption and misappropriation of the limited supplies on hand reduced the soldiers' daily food intake to near starvation levels.

In 1941, the Chinese National Institute of Health wrote that the diet was far less than minimum requirements. The Chinese National Health Administration added that only 40% of the 4.5 million new conscripts were physically fit. They estimated that more than 50% became sick with nutritional or infectious illnesses before they could enroll in the army. In other words, the army could not properly function as the food they were being provided did not adequately meet their bodily standards.

Much as Dr. Erich Mamlok had indicated in his earlier reports, Dr. George Schön wrote of the loss of life due to malnutrition and disease that they observed on the Yichang front in Hubei province on the Yangtze River (Chángjiāng). The 18th Division was the only one receiving the full rations of 680 grams of rice, which every commander received for each registered soldier. In all other divisions, they were not getting more than 567 grams. Only in hospitals were the corrupt practices of kickbacks and bribes reduced due to the fear of weakening the troops. However, even the 454 grams of rice the soldiers were provided was considered quantitatively and qualitatively insufficient as the vegetable protein and vitamins in the rice were completely destroyed by the time the two- to three-year-old rice got to the soldiers. Eventually, the Guomindang's inability to meet the increased nutritional and medical demands imposed by modern warfare and its failure to provide adequate food and public health for the Chinese people became a key factor in its later downfall.

Dietary Conflicts

During World War II, the United States supported China in resisting Japanese aggression and provided military aid. The United States believed that improving the diet of Chinese soldiers, particularly by increasing meat consumption, would enhance their strength and combat effectiveness. However, this plan clashed with China's traditional dietary culture and resource limitations, ultimately failing to achieve the expected results.

To the Western audience, meat was considered a necessary part of a nutritionally strong diet. They argued that, not only was meat essential to Americans, but during World War II, the United States government also elevated meat to a symbol of masculine power. For Americans, ensuring that the Chinese military consumed enough meat was thought to be key to growing Chinese soldiers' power and strength. However, the average Chinese person consumed little to no meat. In fact, most Chinese people primarily ate rice, soybeans, and vegetables, a dietary pattern that many Western observers found difficult to understand.

Research published in the *China Medical Journal*, the official Shanghai-based publication of the Chinese Medical Association in the early 1900s, demonstrated that traditional Chinese foods could provide sufficient nutrition without the need for meat. These studies, published again in English, were intended to help the Western audience understand the dietary differences between the two countries. The findings revealed that soybeans, which were plentiful in China, contained nearly as much protein as meat. Soybeans were not only nutritious but also inexpensive and readily available, making them an ideal source of sustenance, particularly for the impoverished rural population that outnumbered urban dwellers. However, despite the Chinese military demonstrating their resilience and the effectiveness of their diet, save for the portion size, many Americans still believed that China's diet was lackluster.

As a result, the Americans explored various strategies, including increasing vegetable production, long-distance food transportation, and even distributing processed foods. However, increasing vegetable production was a lengthy process, and the lack of proper roads and refrigeration made transportation even more difficult. Additionally, the lack of adequate machinery made food processing impractical. The Americans ultimately concluded that it was their responsibility to provide the necessary supplies for Chinese soldiers as they could not rely on Chinese government agencies to significantly improve the soldiers' conditions. By 1945, the United States had developed a robust distribution system that ensured soldiers received all the necessary supplies, which could be directly delivered to the front lines of anywhere in the world, all coordinated from the industrial center of Chicago. This system, refined during World War I and further improved in the years leading up to World War II, was crucial for maintaining the American military's global supply lines.

Malaria

During the Second Sino-Japanese War, China was ravaged by war while also facing a severe public health crisis. Epidemics such as cholera, plague, malaria, typhoid fever, and dysentery spread rapidly in the midst of conflict and poverty, claiming countless lives. Overcrowded refugee camps, poor sanitary conditions, and an extreme shortage of medical resources turned China into a breeding ground for infectious diseases during the war.

Malaria was one of the most severe infectious diseases in wartime China. In some regions, the infection rate reached as high as 95%, with the disease spreading particularly rampant in Yunnan and Guizhou. Most migrants who moved to the southwestern region had no immunity to malaria, leading to an outbreak of the epidemic. Guizhou, which served as a base for international medical relief teams, recorded approximately eight hundred thousand malaria cases in 1938 alone. Malaria affected nearly all medical personnel of the Chinese Red Cross.

Although the Chinese military attempted to use the locally produced drug Fraxin to treat malaria, its efficacy lacked reliable data. Meanwhile, more effective drugs such as quinine were difficult to distribute widely due to their high cost. The primary preventive measures still relied on mosquito nets and water source management, but these methods were difficult to fully implement in the disruptive wartime environment.

Bacillary Dysentery

Soldiers and civilians on the Yangtze River (Chángjiāng) frontline also faced the threat of bacillary dysentery, an infectious disease caused by bacterial infection. In 1938, an epidemic broke out in Guangdong, Hunan, and Henan. According to reports from the Chinese Red Cross, approximately 20% of the frontline population suffered from bacillary dysentery. Doctors described overcrowded military hospitals where dysentery wards presented heartbreaking scenes: sanitation was nonexistent, feces flowed unchecked across the floors, soldiers huddled together in sleep, unable to escape the stench, and medical staff had to touch bodies to confirm whether their fellow patients had already passed away.

In wartime China, the harsh environment exacerbated the risk of bacterial infection. Even though the Chinese Red Cross produced a substantial amount of sodium sulfate and some emetine hydrochloride for military hospitals stationed in the Wuhan area to treat dysentery, the effectiveness of these drugs was significantly reduced in the absence of proper nutrition and care.

To improve drinking water sanitation on the front lines, the Chinese Red Cross distributed bamboo tubes filled with bleaching powder for soldiers to disinfect their drinking water. However, due to the high cost of disinfection tablets, most soldiers still opted to boil their water before drinking.

Cholera

Cholera, a highly contagious disease transmitted through contaminated food and water, was also mainly caused by the overcrowded conditions and poor sanitation in wartime China. In 1939, a massive cholera outbreak in Guiyang overwhelmed all nearby hospitals. Many patients succumbed to severe dehydration, and corpses piled up along the streets, unable to be buried in time.

The Chinese Red Cross recognized the importance of the cholera vaccine and initially purchased it from French Indochina. However, as Japan's blockade of French Indochina intensified, China began producing its own vaccines. In 1943, the United States Relief Committee estimated that China was producing approximately one million doses of vaccines annually for cholera, typhoid, diphtheria, tetanus, and epidemic typhus, significantly reducing the extent and severity of cholera outbreaks.

The International Medical Teams reported endemic plague outbreaks in Yunnan, Fujian, and Zhejiang. Doctors discovered a large number of sudden deaths in certain villages, along with numerous dead rats, confirming plague outbreaks.

They attempted to implement disease control measures, but the mass exodus of residents from affected areas made epidemic control exceptionally difficult.

Tuberculosis

The harsh wartime conditions caused a sharp rise in tuberculosis mortality rates. With limited sanatoriums and medical resources, many patients had to be treated in makeshift facilities, and late-stage patients had extremely low survival rates. Civilians, soldiers, and workers alike suffered greatly as overcrowded refugee camps and malnutrition created ideal conditions for the disease to spread. Traditional Chinese medicine was often used as an attempt to alleviate symptoms, but without effective treatment, patients were forced to endure the disease and faced grim survival rates. The destruction of cities and hospitals further restricted access to proper healthcare.

Efforts to mitigate the crisis were largely ineffective given the dire circumstances. The makeshift treatment centers were established in repurposed schools and buildings, but these were lacking in many aspects including proper isolation, leading to further spread. Public health campaigns promoted hygiene and fresh air as preventive measures, but such recommendations were difficult to follow amid the chaos of war. Tuberculosis was ultimately one of the deadliest threats of the time, devastating entire communities and leaving a lasting health crisis in its wake.

Sanitation

As a result of infectious disease outbreaks and relapses from poor hygiene, improving environmental sanitation became a core focus of public health agencies. Efforts primarily included well disinfection, waste disposal, pest extermination, and toilet renovations, with well and toilet improvements being the most extensive. Additionally, managing the public food industry and street vendors was a key aspect of hygiene control, as gastrointestinal diseases were widely transmitted through food. Health authorities strengthened regulations on beverages like alcohol, tea, and fruit juices to curb germ spread.

For example, on April 29, 1941, the Sichuan Provincial Health Laboratory's epidemic prevention committee passed the proposal "How to Ban Dining Establishments." By the later wartime period, public dining and street vendor management became more institutionalized. The 1944 "Wartime Health Work Evaluation Standards" required food and fruits to be covered with mosquito nets in summer and subjected to bacterial testing. Since epidemic prevention depended on public awareness, health institutions actively launched campaigns, distributing flyers, organizing health lectures and exhibitions, posting slogans and posters, and promoting health knowledge through newspapers.

During World War II, China's high maternal mortality rate became a widespread concern among professionals. Maternal and child health was regarded as the foundation of national healthcare and thus became a key focus of public health services. According to a 1936 survey, for every one thousand women giving birth during wartime, fifteen died, and for every one thousand newborns, two hundred died, making the mortality rate the highest in the world, even surpassing countries with relatively underdeveloped healthcare systems like India, Egypt, and Poland.

Traditional childbirth methods contributed to this high mortality rate. At the time, untrained relatives often assisted with deliveries, and many women, influenced by feudal beliefs, were too embarrassed to seek medical help, even in dangerous situations. Reports from the Ning County Health Center detailed how many women delivered while squatting on the ground, using their teeth to cut the umbilical cord, simply tying it with cloth, and considering the delivery complete after a brief cleaning. To address this, government agencies vigorously promoted modern childbirth methods, including prenatal examinations, professional delivery services, postnatal care, and related educational programs. Prenatal exams were particularly emphasized, as they could prevent complications such as difficult deliveries, premature births, and stillbirths. Statistics show that areas adopting aseptic delivery methods saw a significant decline in both infant and maternal mortality rates.

Meanwhile, the war severely affected students' health, with government health checks revealing that over ninety percent of students had health issues, and very few were in good physical and mental condition. Recognizing the importance of student health for national development, the Guomindang prioritized school hygiene. A 1940 record from a health institute noted that after health checks, the institute immediately began treatment and assigned personnel to visit schools weekly to treat trachoma, skin diseases, and eye-ear issues. For urgent cases, students were referred to hospitals and granted free registration privileges. Since schools lacked sufficient first-aid kits due to limited medical resources, health institutes set up mobile public health medicine kits, rotating them among schools. For health education, hygiene knowledge materials were compiled and provided to teachers for instruction. Among various school health measures, student health checks were the most common. Given the wartime economic difficulties, the government struggled to implement high-cost medical programs, but health checks required no additional expenses and effectively monitored students' health. Except for 1941, when Japanese air raids caused large-scale student migration, the number of students examined increased by 133.5% between 1942 and 1943.

Hospitals themselves were also ill-equipped with proper sanitation supplies and medical resources. Many field hospitals were set up in makeshift facilities such as schools, temples, warehouses, or even tents. They were only hospitals by name. To reduce infections, these hospitals categorized patients based on injury severity and disease type, such as severe injury wards, minor injury wards, and infectious disease wards. Due to construction limitations, hospital windows and doors were often left open to improve ventilation and slow bacterial growth.

Disinfection and epidemic prevention were critical, but resources were scarce. Surgical instruments like scalpels, tweezers, and scissors were typically sterilized with alcohol, boiling water, or iodine, but due to shortages, they were often reused, increasing infection risks. Bed linens and blankets, rarely replaced due to supply shortages, became breeding grounds for lice and fleas. To mitigate this, medical staff periodically exposed sheets to sunlight and disinfected them with lime or sulfur. Hospital floors were usually cleaned with lime water, and sulfur or bleaching powder was burned in patient rooms for air disinfection.

Surgical and wound treatment conditions were equally dire. Field surgeries were conducted in rudimentary rooms or tents, with operating tables made from wooden boards or metal frames covered with coarse cloth or newspaper. With disinfectants like iodine, carbolic acid, and bleaching powder in short supply, some hospitals had to substitute with hot water or alcohol, making sterile procedures nearly impossible. Doctors and nurses often had to reuse gloves or operate bare-handed, greatly increasing infection risks. To combat bacterial infections in wounds, hospitals used sulfa drugs and disinfected with alcohol or iodine. However, with limited bandages and cotton, many soldiers had to use reused bandages, cloth strips, or even newspapers, leading to gangrene and septicemia, which resulted in extremely high mortality rates.

Another aspect of dirtiness that led to the rapid spread of infectious diseases was the poorly sanitized food and water sources. To mitigate this, hospitals disinfected water sources with lime or bleaching powder and instructed patients to drink boiled water. Highly contagious diseases were managed through isolation wards, and medical staff were required to disinfect their hands with bleach or alcohol after patient contact, though shortages of soap and disinfectants often forced them to wash with hot water instead.

These wartime medical experiences played a crucial role in shaping China's public health system after the war. Involvement of different teams and programs such as International Medical Relief Corps, the Chinese Red Cross, and health-focused programs in the battlefield during wartime China marked a major shift in attitudes toward human life in war. By establishing hospitals—even shabby, makeshift ones—and introducing epidemic prevention measures, these organizations set a precedent for organized medical relief in China. Their abilities to mobilize both national and international resources solidified its role in China's medical and humanitarian landscape, influencing modern medical relief efforts and shaping the future of humanitarian aid in China and beyond.

戰地工作
與生活環境

營養不良

二戰期間，相較於西方國家，中國仍是一個相對貧困的農業經濟體，難以滿足其超過五億人口的基本飲食需求。中國人民的營養狀況本已嚴峻，加之外援物資受到嚴格禁運、現代戰爭帶來的毀滅性破壞，以及接連不斷的乾旱，使得情況雪上加霜。普遍的營養不良與飢荒，成為阻礙基本醫療服務推行的核心難題。

多位國際醫療救護隊醫師曾記錄下中國戰時營養不良的嚴重情況。在 1939 年紅十字會第 32 救護隊[1]的一份報告中，德國醫師孟樂克（Dr. Erich Mamlok）指出：「由於大多數病患長期營養不良，醫療工作變得更加困難。由吳醫師在軍方特別許可下進行的驗屍結果顯示，幾乎每一具遺體都有慢性營養不良的跡象，包括沒有皮下脂肪與網膜脂肪、貧血、腸道萎縮、骨骼軟化等。有些腸炎個案中，腸道發炎極其輕微，患者實際死因很可能是營養不良而非腸炎本身。這類營養缺乏主要是蛋白質（尤其是白蛋白）和維生素等必要營養素的不足。」

中國紅十字會估計，政府每日提供給中國軍隊的軍糧配給為：米 953 克、蔬菜 273 克、豬油 10 克與食鹽 13 克。這意味著士兵們每天僅靠兩餐維生，內容通常是一碟蔬菜配些許肉類，或更常見的是清湯、白米飯與米湯粥。更糟的是，有限的物資經常遭到貪污或挪用，使得士兵每日實際攝取的食物量少的可憐，長期處於營養不良的狀態。

1941 年，中國中央衛生實驗院[2]指出，當時軍糧的營養遠低於最低所需標準。衛生署進一步補充道，450 萬名新徵召的士兵中，僅有約 40% 符合基本體能要求。該單位估計，超過半數的新兵在入伍前便因營養不良或傳染病而體質羸弱。換言之，軍隊無法正常運作的根本原因之一，在於士兵所獲得的糧食無法滿足其基本生理需求。

正如孟樂克在前述報告中所指出的，沈恩醫生也在瀕臨長江的湖北

---

[1] 孟樂克醫生是中國紅十字會的僱員。

[2] https://reurl.cc/0KldA9

省宜昌前線地區，記錄了他們所觀察到的因營養不良與疾病導致的大量死亡情況。第十八師是唯一獲得完整口糧的部隊，每名登記在案的士兵配給 680 克白米，由各級指揮官統一領取。而在其他師部，實際配發量往往不超過 567 克。唯有在醫院內，因擔心削弱軍力，回扣與賄賂等腐敗現象才沒那麼嚴重。然而，即使是實際提供的 454 克白米，從質與量上都遠遠不足。這些白米因儲存已久（通常為兩至三年），其中所含的植物蛋白與維生素早已遭到破壞。

飲食文化的衝突

在第二次世界大戰期間，美國為協助中國抵抗日本的侵略，向中國提供軍事援助。美方認為，改善中國士兵的飲食，特別是提高肉類攝取量，能夠增強體力與戰鬥力。然而，這項計畫與中國傳統的飲食文化以及當時資源匱乏的現實情況產生衝突，最終未能達成預期成效。

對西方人而言，肉類被視為營養充足飲食中不可或缺的一部分。他們主張，不僅對美國人來說肉類至關重要，在第二次世界大戰期間，美國政府更將肉類提升為陽剛力量的象徵。美國人認為，提升中國士兵力量與體能的關鍵，就是要確保軍隊攝取足夠的肉類。然而，一般中國人平時幾乎不食用肉類。事實上，大多數中國人以米飯、大豆和蔬菜為主食，這種飲食模式讓許多西方人難以理解。

根據發表於《中華醫學雜誌》的研究顯示，傳統中式飲食方式在不依賴肉類的情況下，同樣能提供充足的營養。該期刊是中華醫學會在 1915 年於上海創辦的官方出版物，這些研究後來也以英文刊出，旨在幫助西方讀者理解中西飲食文化的差異。研究發現，在中國極為普遍的大豆，也含有幾乎可以媲美肉類的豐富蛋白質。大豆不僅營養豐富，還價格低廉、取得容易，特別適合作為主食來源，尤其對於人口遠多於城市居民的貧困農村地區而言更是如此。然而，儘管中國軍隊展現出強韌的體魄，實際上也顯示其飲食方式是有效的（除了份量較少之外），許多美國人仍認為中國的飲食缺乏營養，不盡如人意。

因此，美國人嘗試了多種策略，包括增加蔬菜產量、進行長途糧食運輸，甚至分發加工食品。然而，增加蔬菜產量是一個漫長的過程，而缺乏適當的道路與冷藏設施又讓運輸困難重重。此外，由於機械設備不足，加工食品的生產也變得不切實際。最終，美方得出結論：他們必須自行提供中國士兵所需的補給，因為無法依賴中國政府機構顯著改善士兵的生活條件。到了1945年，美國已建立起一套穩健的配送體系，能將所有必要物資直接送達世界任何地點的前線，而這一切的調度工作皆以芝加哥的工業中心為核心。這套系統最初於第一次世界大戰期間建立，並在二戰前進一步優化，成為維繫美軍全球供應鏈的關鍵基礎。

瘧疾

在抗日戰爭期間，中國不僅深陷戰火，同時也面臨嚴峻的公共衛生危機。霍亂、鼠疫、瘧疾、傷寒與痢疾等傳染病在戰亂與貧困之中迅速蔓延，奪走無數生命。擁擠的難民營、惡劣的衛生條件，以及醫療資源的極度匱乏，使得戰時中國成為傳染病滋生的溫床。

瘧疾是當時最為嚴重的傳染病之一。在某些地區，感染率高達95%，其中又以雲南與貴州最為嚴重。大多數遷徙至中國西南地區的移民對瘧疾毫無免疫力，因而引發大規模疫情。貴州是眾多國際醫療救援隊的駐紮基地，在1938年即記錄了約八十萬例瘧疾病例。瘧疾幾乎影響了中國紅十字會所有的醫療人員。

儘管中國軍方試圖使用國產藥物「秦皮苷」（Fraxin，由白蠟樹提煉而成）治療瘧疾，但其療效缺乏可靠數據支持。與此同時，效果較佳的藥物如奎寧（quinine），因價格高昂難以廣泛分發。當時的主要預防手段仍然仰賴蚊帳與水源管理，但這些方法在戰時動盪的環境下難以全面實施。

桿菌性痢疾

長江戰線上的軍民也面臨桿菌性痢疾的威脅，這是一種由細菌感染引起的傳染病。1938 年，廣東、湖南與河南爆發痢疾疫情。根據中國紅十字會的報告，前線約有 20% 的人口罹患桿菌性痢疾。根據醫生描述，軍醫院人滿為患，痢疾病房情況淒慘：衛生條件極差，排泄物橫流於地，士兵擠在一起睡覺，臭氣熏天。醫護人員甚至需要透過觸碰病患的身體，以確認他們是否已經去世。

戰時中國的惡劣環境進一步加劇了細菌感染的風險。雖然中國紅十字會曾為駐守武漢地區的軍醫院製造大量硫酸鈉與少量鹽酸吐根鹼，以治療痢疾，但在缺乏營養與妥善照護的情況下，這些藥物的療效大打折扣。

為改善前線飲用水衛生，中國紅十字會曾發放裝有漂白粉的竹筒，供士兵消毒飲用水。然而，由於消毒藥片價格昂貴，多數士兵仍選擇僅將水煮沸後飲用。

霍亂

霍亂是一種透過受污染食物與水源傳播的高度傳染性疾病，戰時中國擁擠的生活環境與惡劣的公共衛生條件也成為主要致病因素。1939 年，貴陽爆發大規模霍亂疫情，當地所有醫院皆無法應對，大量患者因嚴重脫水死亡，街頭上堆滿了無法及時掩埋的屍體。

中國紅十字會意識到霍亂疫苗的重要性後，初期自法屬印度支那進口疫苗，但隨著日本對法屬印度支那的封鎖日益嚴峻，中國開始自行生產疫苗。1943 年，美國醫藥助華會估計，中國每年約生產一百萬劑霍亂、傷寒、白喉、破傷風與流行性斑疹傷寒等疫苗，成功降低霍亂疫情的範圍與嚴重程度。

國際醫療隊也回報，雲南、福建與浙江等地出現地方性鼠疫疫情。醫生在部分村莊發現大量居民猝死，並發現許多鼠屍，確認為鼠疫爆發。雖然當地嘗試實施防疫措施，但因大量居民逃離疫區，使得疫情難以控制。

肺結核

　　嚴酷的戰爭環境導致肺結核死亡率大幅上升。由於療養院與醫療資源極為有限，許多患者只能在臨時搭建的設施中接受治療，而末期患者的存活率極低。無論是平民、士兵還是勞工，都深受其害，擁擠的難民營與普遍的營養不良，為肺結核的蔓延提供了溫床。當時多以中藥試圖緩解症狀，但由於缺乏真正有效的治療方法，患者往往只能忍受病痛折磨，存活率更是慘不忍睹。城市與醫院的毀壞，也進一步限制了民眾得到正規醫療服務的機會。

　　儘管當時的政府試圖控制疫情，但在如此艱困的情況下，成效極為有限。許多臨時醫療處所設在學校與各類建築中，然而這些地方往往缺乏完善的隔離措施，反而促使疫情進一步擴散。雖然衛生單位大力宣傳公共衛生，鼓勵民眾保持清潔與多接觸新鮮空氣以預防感染，但在戰亂中，這些建議實際上很難落實。肺結核最終成為當時最致命的疾病之一，重創無數社區，並在戰後留下長遠的公共衛生危機。

戰時衛生

　　由於傳染病爆發與惡劣衛生條件引發的疫情反覆，改善環境衛生成為公共衛生機構的核心目標。主要措施包括井水消毒、廢棄物處理、消除蟲害與鼠害，還有整修廁所，其中以井水與廁所改建規模最廣。此外，管理公共飲食業與路邊小販亦是衛生防疫的重要部分，因為腸胃道疾病多經由食物傳播。當局也加強對酒類、茶水與果汁等飲品的管控，以防細菌蔓延。例如，1941年4月29日，四川省衛生實驗處防疫委員會通過「如何取締飲食店及食物」提案。

　　戰爭後期，公共餐飲與路邊攤販管理逐漸制度化，1944年的《戰時衛生工作評判標準》規定夏季食物與水果需用蚊帳覆蓋，並進行細菌檢驗。由於防疫成效取決於民眾的防疫觀念，衛生單位積極展開宣導活動，發放傳單、舉辦衛生講座與展覽，張貼標語與海報，並透過報紙普及衛生知識。

抗戰期間，中國產婦的高死亡率成為醫界普遍關注的問題。醫界視母嬰保健為國民健康基礎，也是公共衛生服務的重要工作。據 1936 年統計，戰時每千名產婦死亡十五人，每千名新生兒死亡兩百人，死亡率居世界之冠，甚至超越當時醫療較落後的印度、埃及與波蘭。

傳統接生方式是造成高死亡率的主因。當時多由缺乏專業訓練的親屬協助分娩，且受封建觀念影響，許多婦女即使危及生命也羞於就醫。寧縣衛生院的報告記載，產婦多蹲地生產，以牙齒咬斷臍帶後簡單用布條綁住傷口，略作清洗便告完成。為改善情況，政府積極推行現代化接生方式，包括產前檢查、專業接生、產後護理及衛生教育。尤重於產前檢查，藉以預防難產、早產與死胎等併發症。統計顯示，採行無菌接生方式的地區，產婦與嬰兒死亡率大幅下降。

同時，戰爭亦嚴重影響學生健康，根據政府體檢的報告顯示，九成以上學生有健康問題，身心健康都良好的幾乎沒有。國民政府意識到學生健康對國家發展的重要性，於是將校園衛生視為重點。1940 年某衛生機構記錄指出，為學生體檢後，機構立即展開治療行動，並每週派員至學校治療沙眼、皮膚病與眼耳疾患，急重病例則轉送醫院並免收掛號費。由於醫療資源匱乏，學校多沒有足夠的急救箱，衛生機構設置流動醫藥箱，輪流派送各校。衛生教育方面，則編寫衛生知識教材供教師授課。其中，因戰時經濟困難，政府難以推行高成本的醫療政策，而體檢不需額外支出，卻能有效關心學生健康狀況，學生體檢因此成為最常見的醫療措施。除 1941 年日軍空襲導致大批學生遷徙外，1942 至 1943 年間，受檢學生人數成長了 133.5%。

由於醫院缺乏衛生用品與醫療資源。許多野戰醫院設於學校、寺廟、倉庫甚至帳篷內，名為醫院，實則簡陋。為防止交叉感染，醫院依傷情及病種分類設立重傷、輕傷和傳染病病房。因建築條件有限，多半敞開窗門以通風抑菌。

消毒與防疫極為重要，但相關資源嚴重匱乏。需使用酒精、沸水或碘酒消毒的手術器械如手術刀、鑷子與剪刀，在物資不足時只能重複使用，大大增加了感染風險。病床鋪蓋極少更換，成為蝨子與跳蚤孳生的溫床，醫護人員會定期在陽光下曝曬床單，或以石灰、硫磺消毒。地面多以石灰水擦拭，病房則燃燒硫磺或漂白粉消毒空氣。

處理手術與傷口的環境極為惡劣。野戰手術多在簡陋的房舍或帳篷內進行，手術台以木板或金屬架鋪布、報紙代替。因碘酒、苯酚（石炭酸）、漂白粉等消毒劑短缺，只能用熱水或酒精代替，無法達成無菌效果。醫護常需重複使用手套，甚至徒手進行手術，感染風險極高。為抑制細菌感染，醫院施用磺胺藥、酒精與碘酒。因繃帶與棉花短缺，士兵常以舊繃帶、布條或報紙包紮，易導致壞疽與敗血症，死亡率極高。

不潔的食品與飲用水亦是疾病快速蔓延的主因。為改善此情況，醫院多以石灰或漂白粉消毒水源，並要求患者飲用煮沸水。高傳染性疾病患者則施以隔離治療，醫護接觸患者後需以漂白水或酒精消毒雙手，惟肥皂與消毒劑匱乏，只能以熱水代替。

這些戰爭時期的醫療經驗，對戰後中國公共衛生體系的建立產生了重要影響。國際醫療救護隊、中國紅十字會及各種衛生組織參與戰時中國醫療救護，改變了過去人命在戰爭中的價值觀。即便僅是破舊的臨時醫院與簡易的防疫措施，也為中國組織性醫療救援立下典範，動員國內外資源和人力，以確保醫療與人道救援的重要地位，對戰後中國乃至全球的人道醫療援助產生深遠影響。

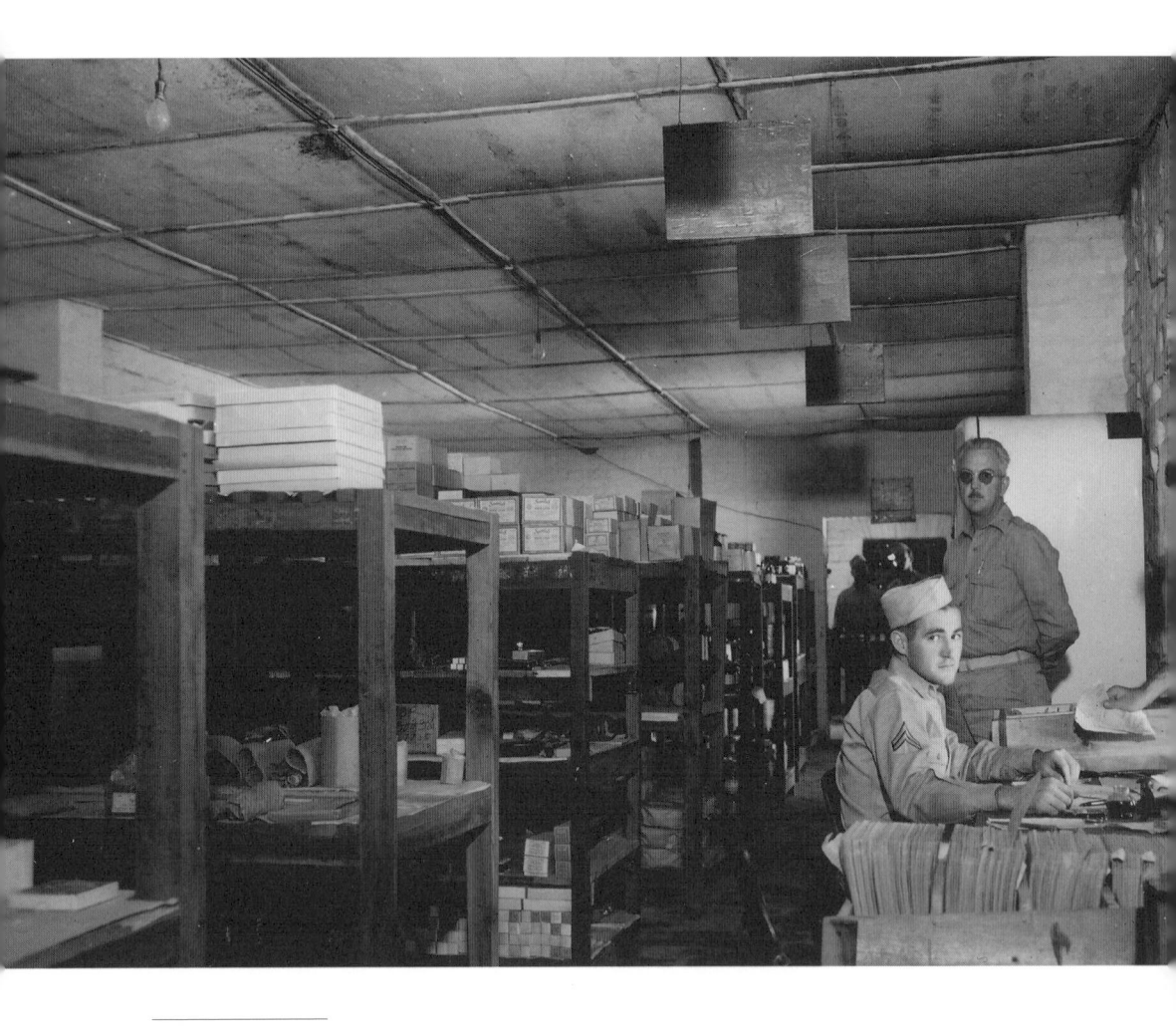

The supply room of the United States 371st Station Hospital.
美軍第 371 駐紮地醫院的物資室。

Date of Photo 時間：December 10, 1944
Credits 來源：美國國家檔案館 Photo Courtesy of National Archives

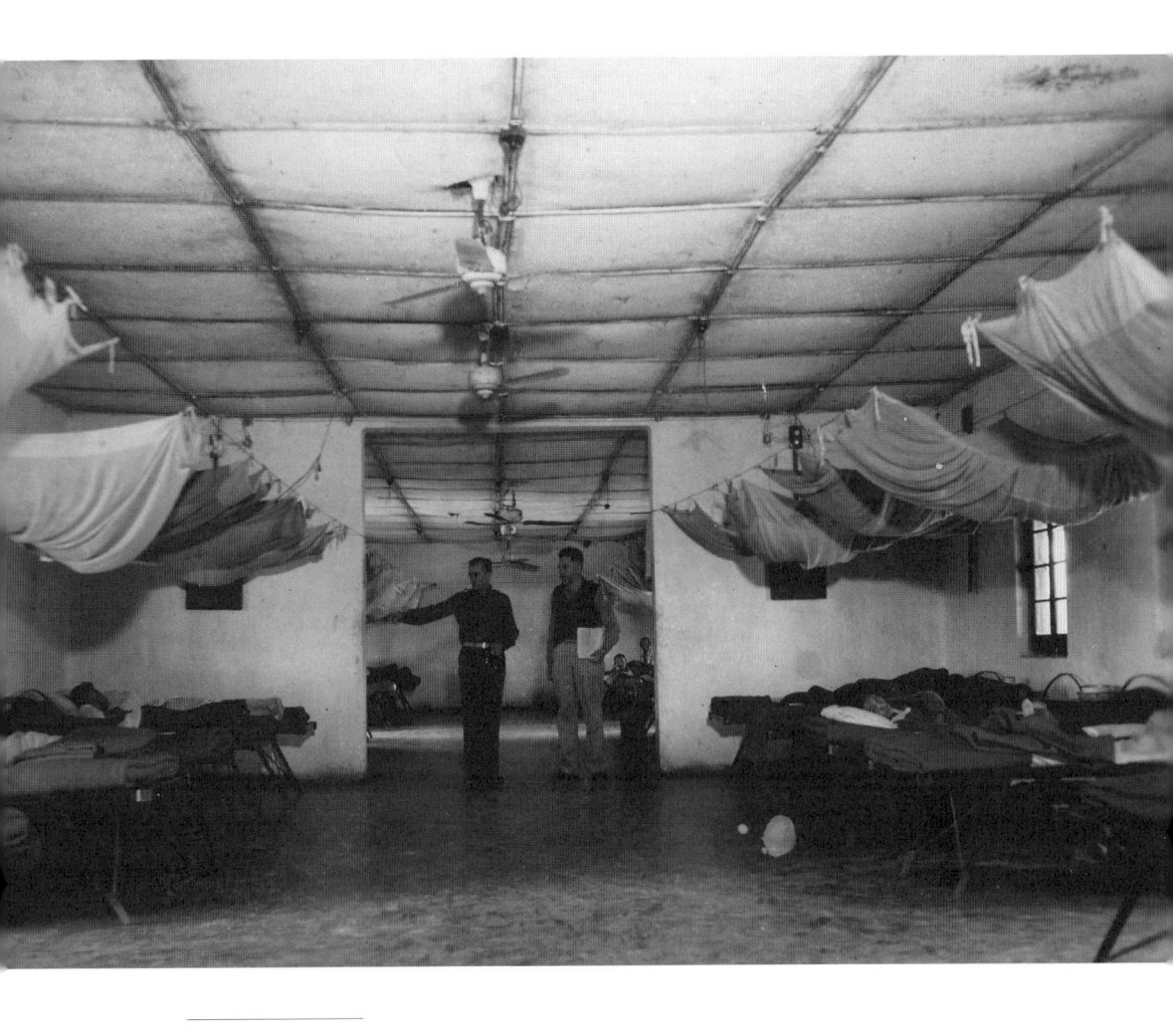

The Chinese Ward United States 371st Station Hospital, Ramgarh India.

美軍第 371 駐紮地醫院中提供給中國病患的病房,位於印度蘭姆伽。

Date of Photo 時間:December 10, 1944
Credits 來源:美國國家檔案館 Photo Courtesy of National Archives

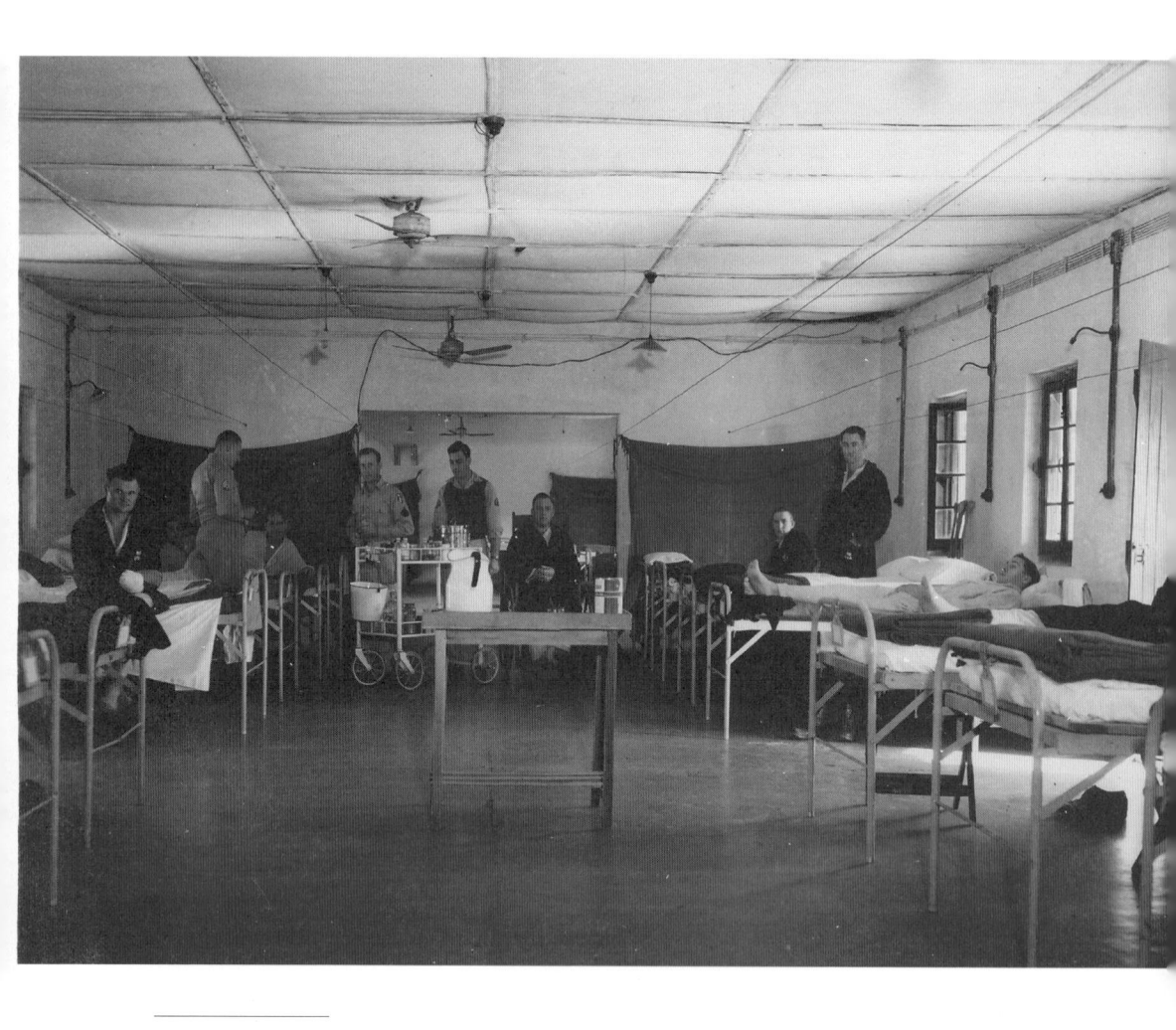

Enlisted personnel and patients in American Ward No.2 of the United States 371st Station Hospital, Ramgarh India.

美軍第 371 駐紮地醫院中第二美國病房的醫療人員和病人，位於印度蘭姆伽。

Date of Photo 時間：December 10, 1944
Credits 來源：美國國家檔案館 Photo Courtesy of National Archives

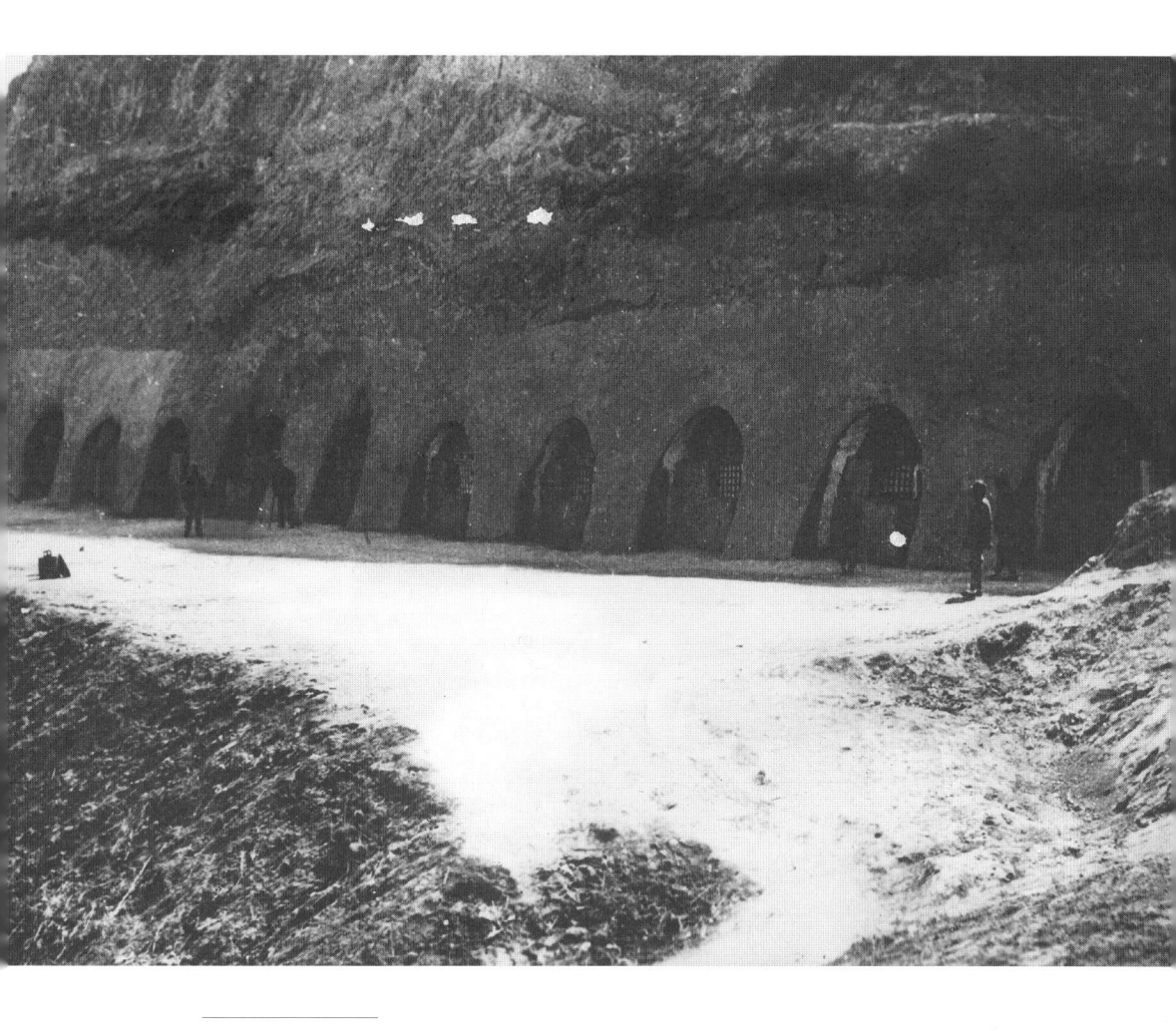

The International Peace Hospital in China Shanxi province, with its solid earth roof, made this hospital one of the safest in China.

中國山西省的國際和平醫院,堅固的土質屋頂使這座醫院成為戰時中國最安全的醫院之一。

Date of Photo 時間:May 25, 1943
Credits 來源:美國國家檔案館 Photo Courtesy of National Archives

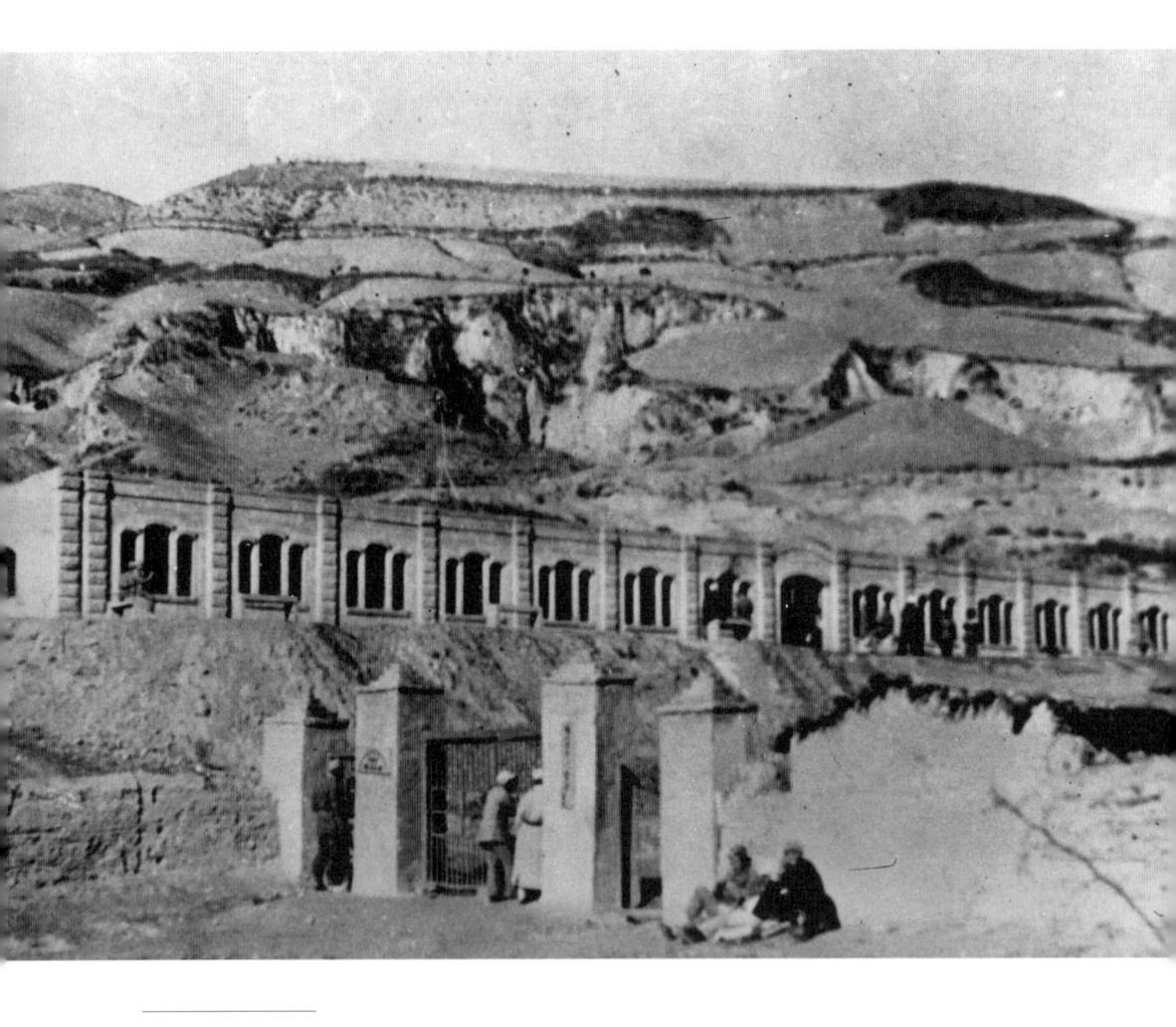

A Canadian-American International Peace Hospital located in China's Shanxi province.

加美國際和平醫院，位於中國山西省。

Date of Photo 時間：不詳 N/A
Credits 來源：美國國家檔案館 Photo Courtesy of National Archives

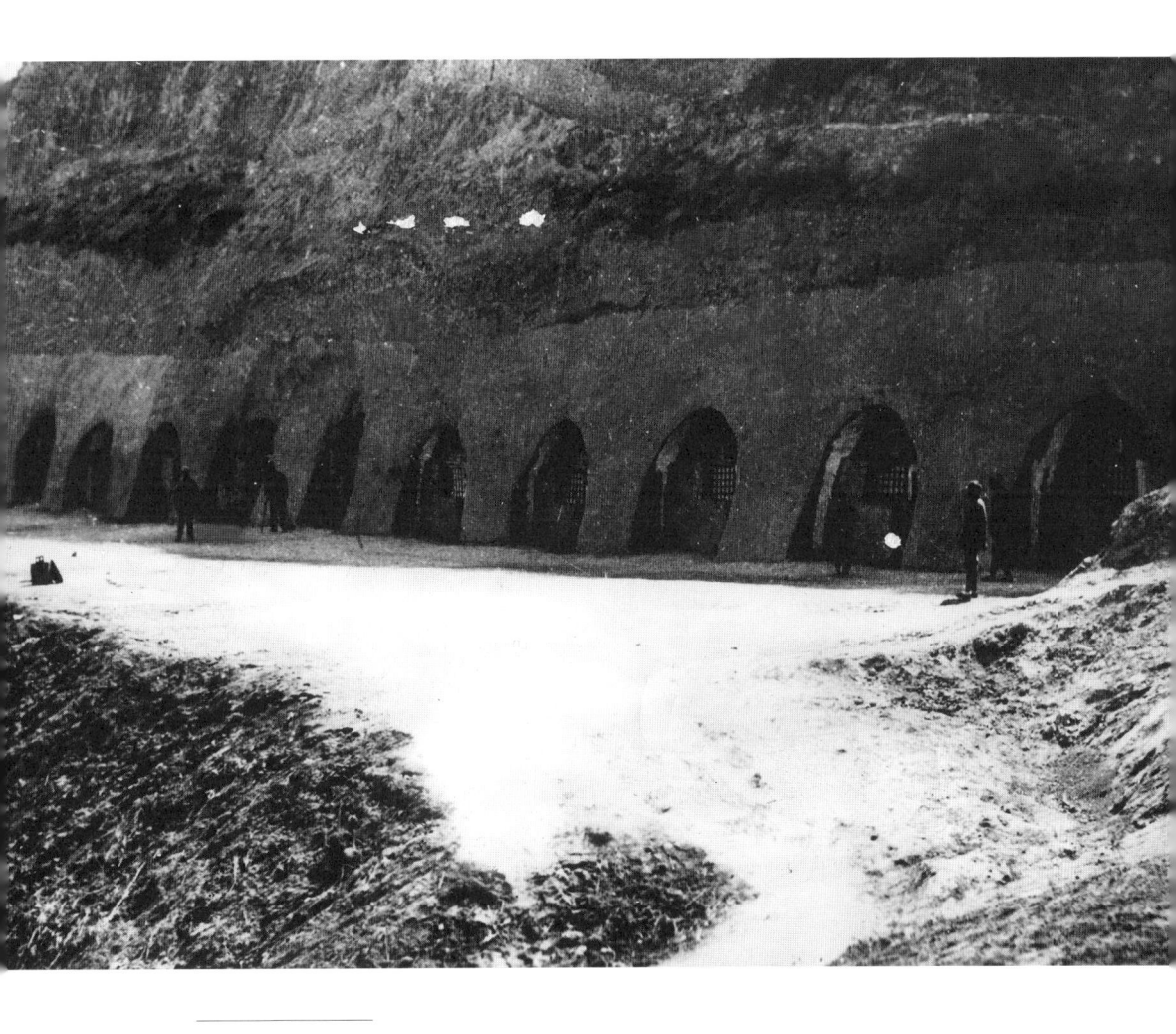

The first floor of the Canadian-American International Peace Hospital in Shanxi Province, despite being repeatedly bombed, was extremely safe as it was carved out of the side of the mountain.

位於山西省的加美國際和平醫院一樓。儘管曾多次遭到轟炸,但因為依山而建,依然十分安穩。

Date of Photo 時間:不詳 N/A
Credits 來源:美國國家檔案館 Photo Courtesy of National Archives

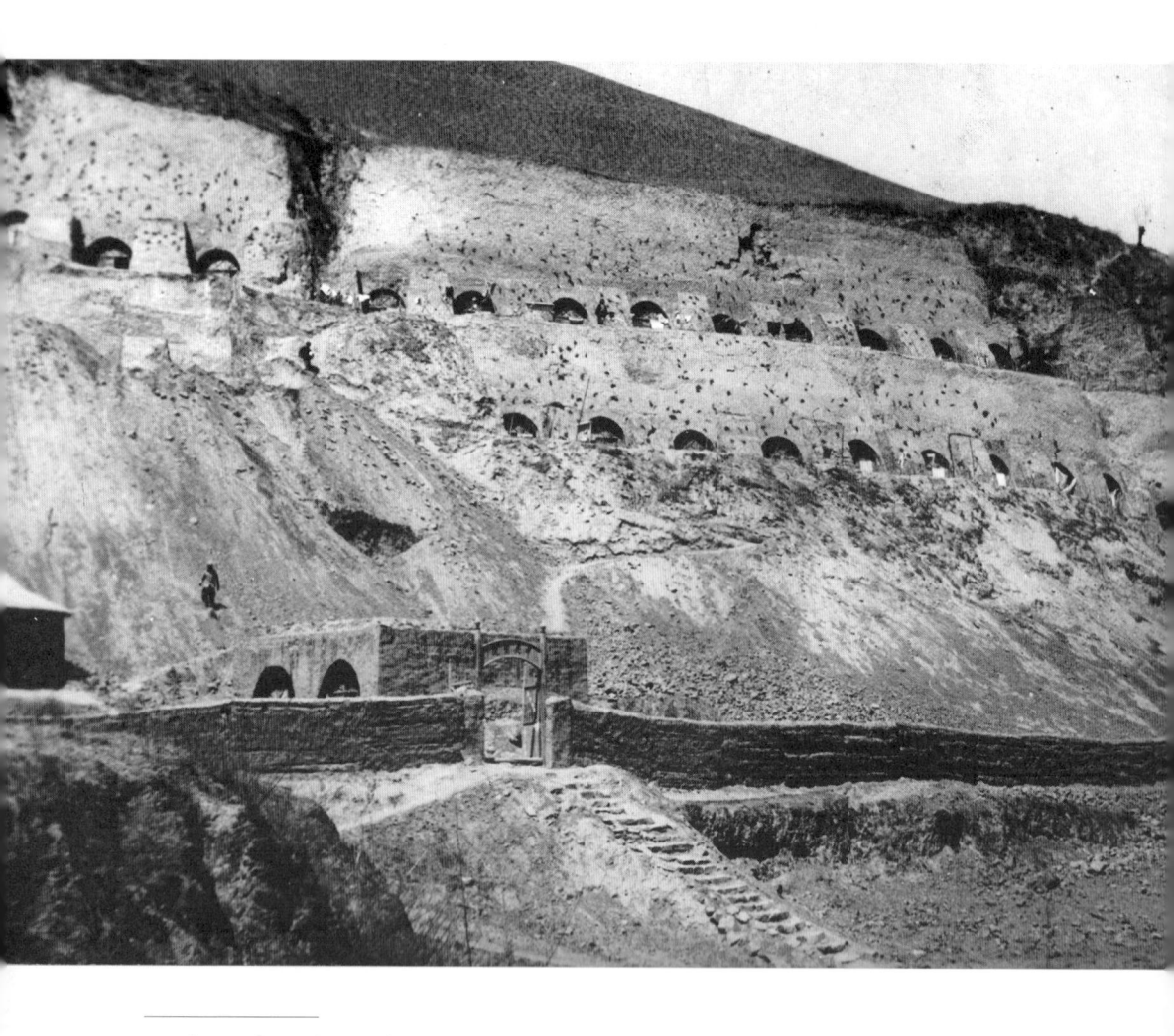

Bomb-proof cave houses from Canadian-American International Peace Hospital in Shanxi Province.

加美國際和平醫院的防空洞,位於山西省。

Date of Photo 時間:不詳 N/A
Credits 來源:美國國家檔案館 Photo Courtesy of National Archives

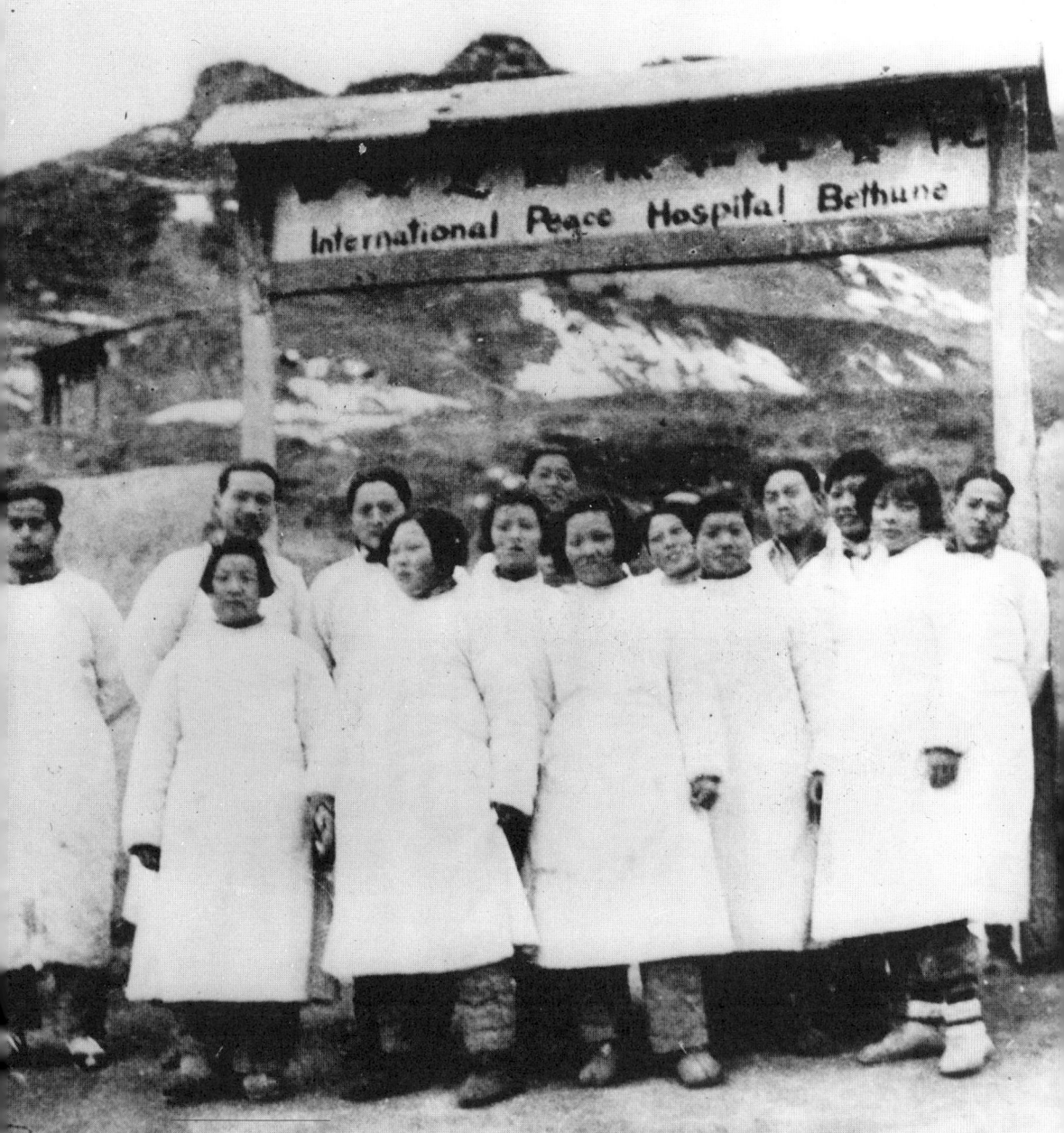

Members of the International Medical Relief Corps standing before the International Peace Hospital.

站在白求恩國際和平醫院前面的國際醫療救護隊隊員們。

Date of Photo 時間：不詳 N/A
Credits 來源：美國國家檔案館 Photo Courtesy of National Archives

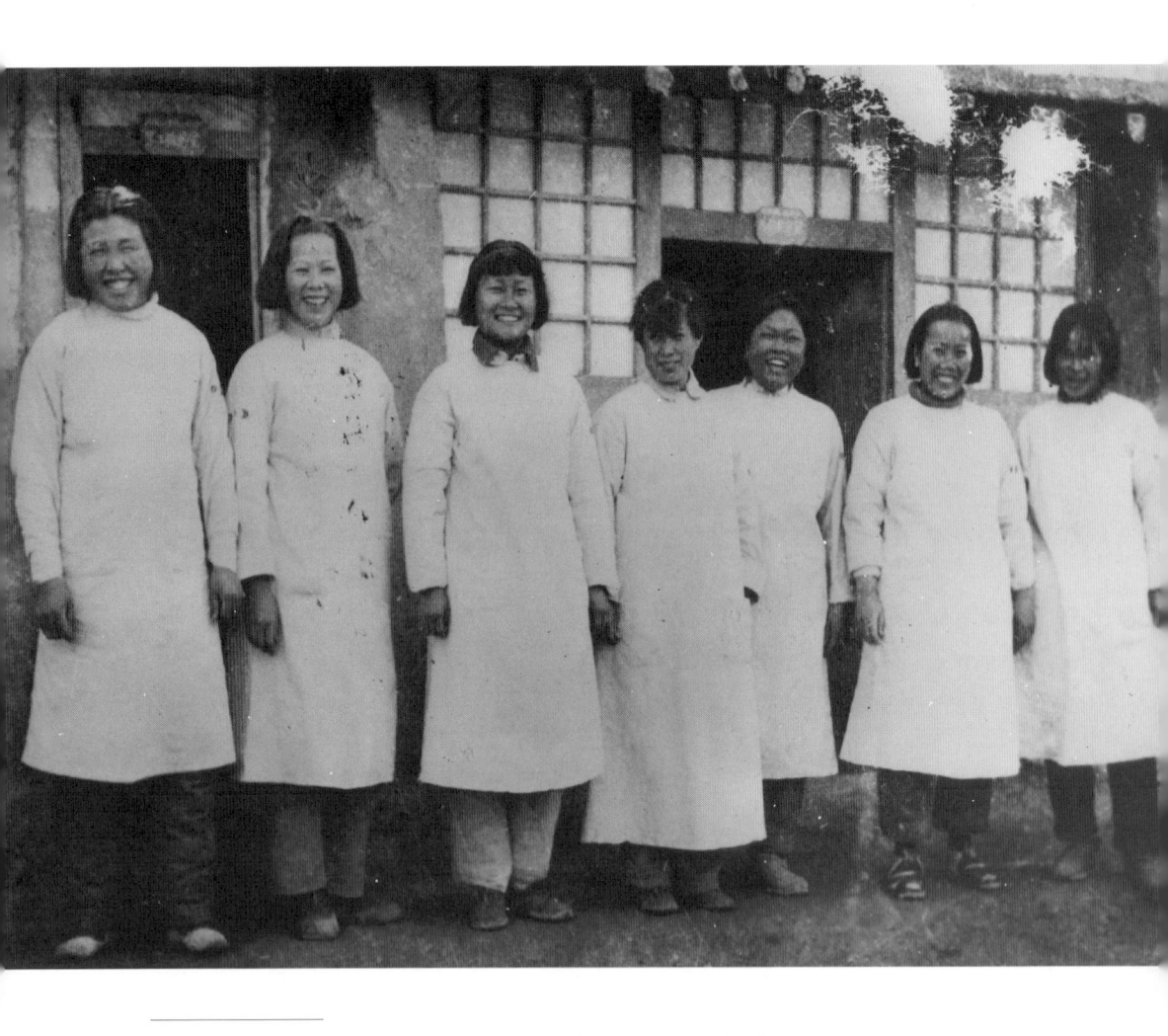

Dr. Basu, a member of the Indian National Congress Medical Mission to China, wrote about the outstanding spirit of unity among a group of nurses at the International Peace Hospital after his visit in 1942.

印度國大黨醫療代表團成員巴蘇博士在 1942 年參訪國際和平醫院後,為該院護理人員之間卓越的團結精神留下文字紀錄。

Date of Photo 時間:不詳 N/A
Credits 來源:美國國家檔案館 Photo Courtesy of National Archives

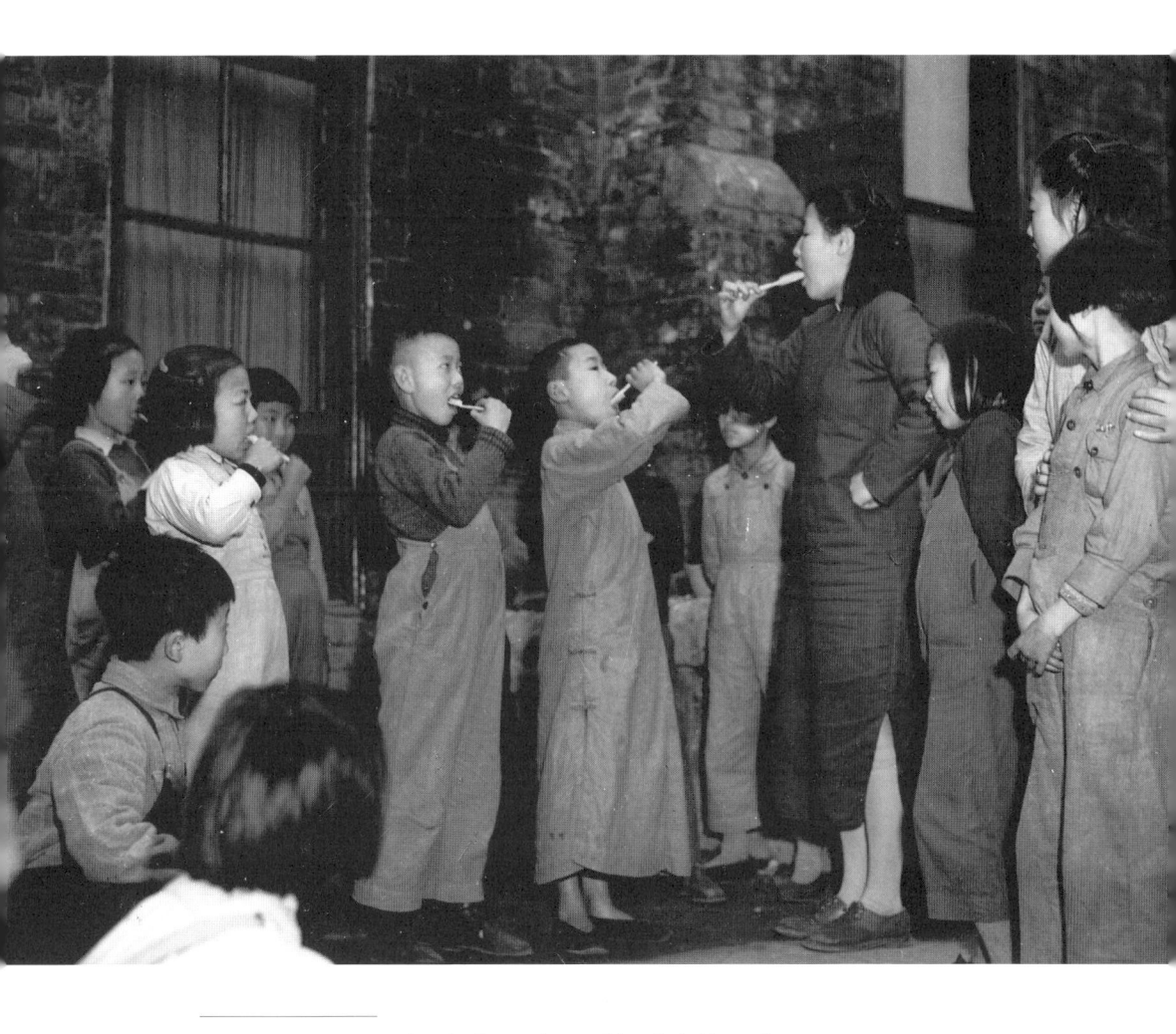

The China Nutritional Aid Clinic educated local children about the importance of brushing their teeth.

援華組織 China Nutritional Aid Clinic 正在教育中國兒童有關刷牙的重要性

Date of Photo 時間：不詳 N/A
Credits 來源：美國國家檔案館 Photo Courtesy of National Archives

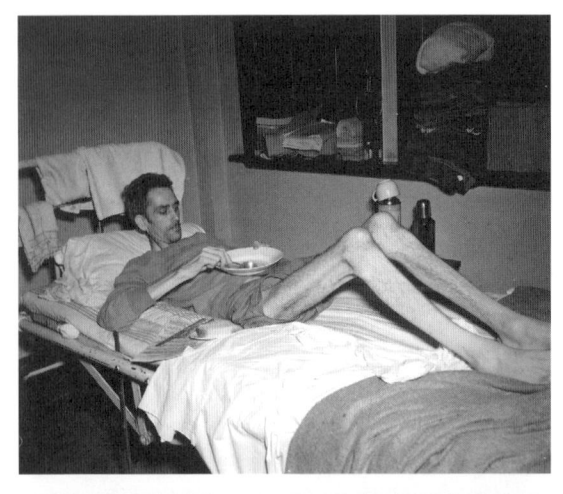

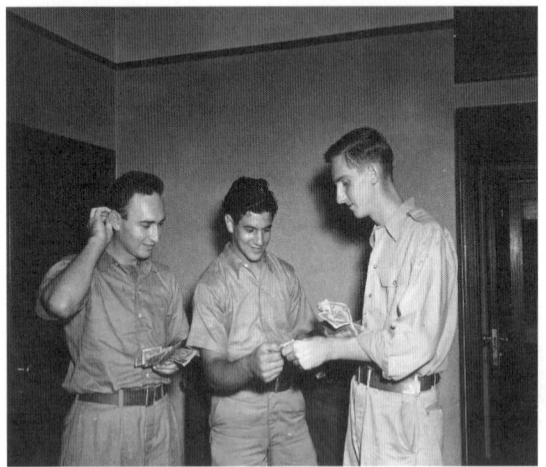

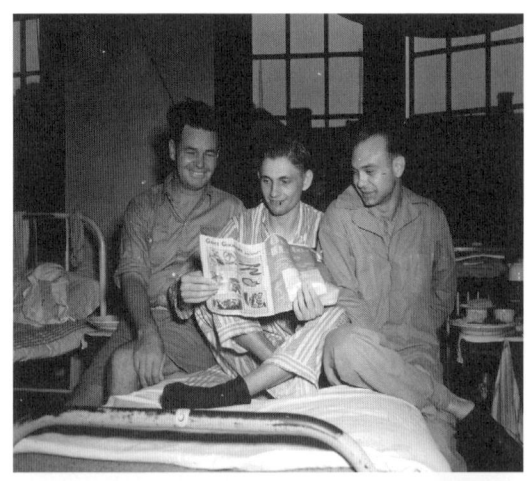

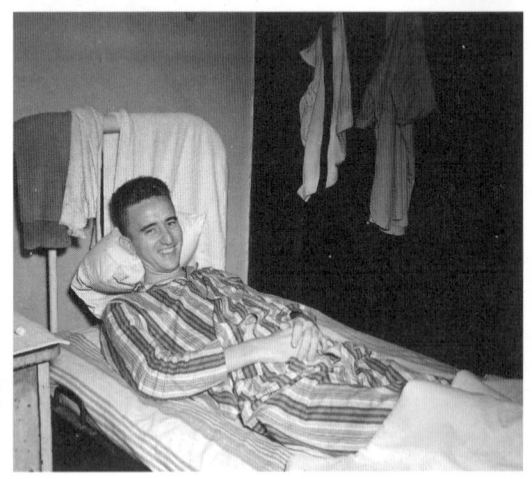

Liberation of American prisoners receiving treatment at St. Luke's Hospital in Shanghai, China.

獲救的美國戰俘在中國上海同仁醫院接受治療。

Date of Photo 時間：October 9, 1945
Credits 來源：美國國家檔案館 Photo Courtesy of National Archives

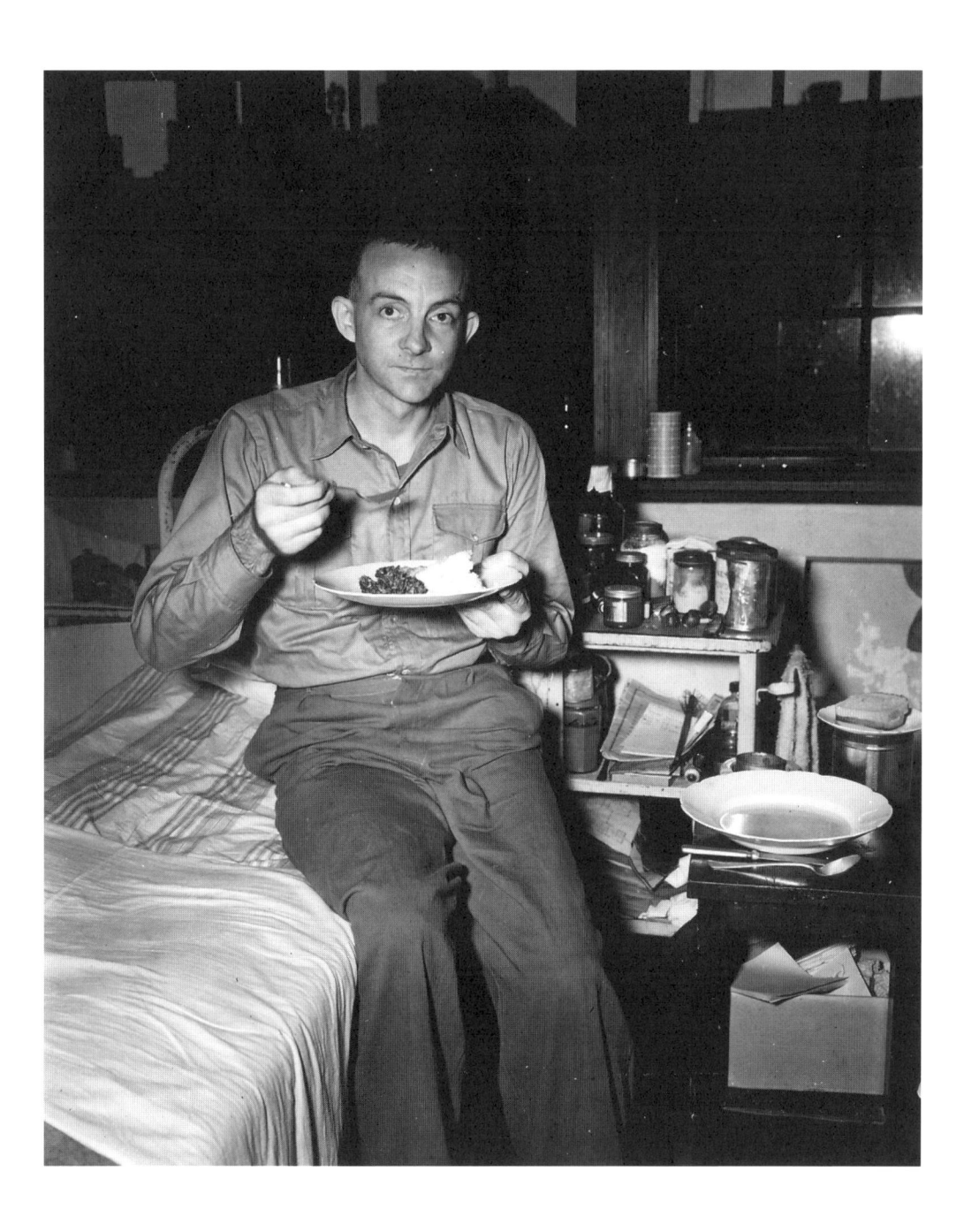

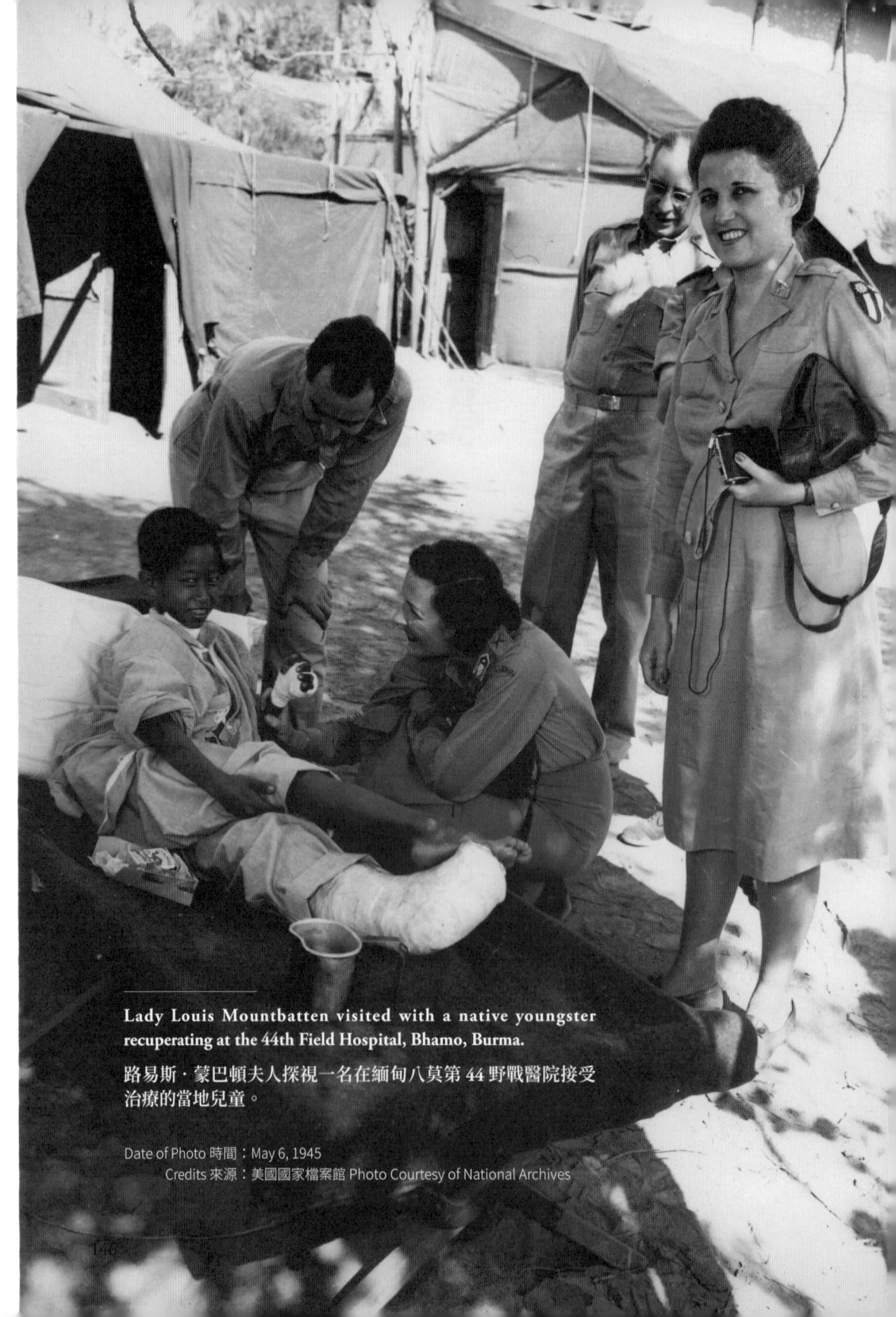

Lady Louis Mountbatten visited with a native youngster recuperating at the 44th Field Hospital, Bhamo, Burma.

路易斯・蒙巴頓夫人探視一名在緬甸八莫第 44 野戰醫院接受治療的當地兒童。

Date of Photo 時間：May 6, 1945
Credits 來源：美國國家檔案館 Photo Courtesy of National Archives

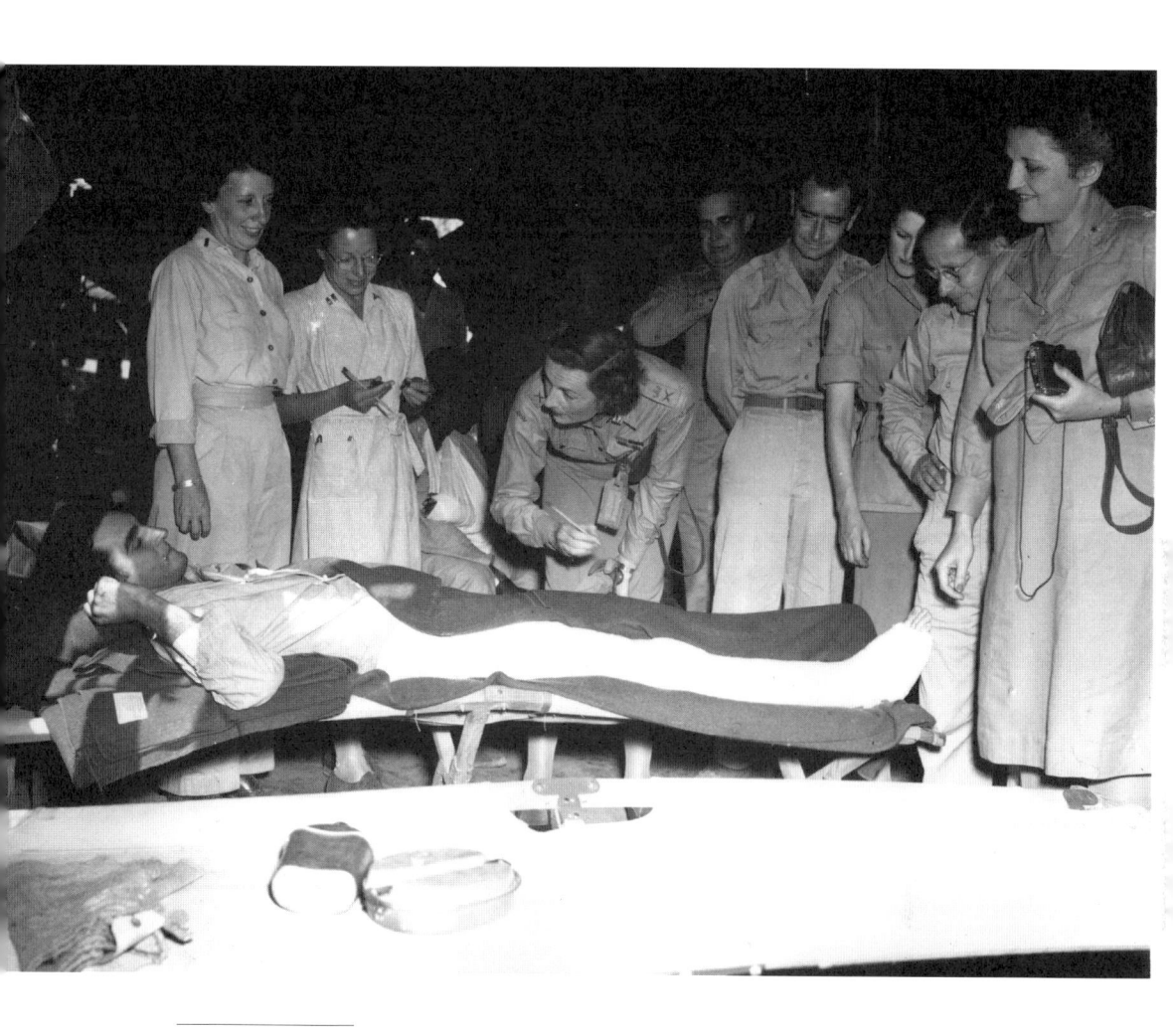

Lady Louis Mountbatten signed her autograph on a plaster cast of a patient in the 44th Field Hospital during her visit to Bhamo, Burma.

路易斯・蒙巴頓夫人訪視緬甸八莫時,在第 44 野戰醫院為一名病患在石膏上簽名。

Date of Photo 時間:May 6, 1945
Credits 來源:美國國家檔案館 Photo Courtesy of National Archives

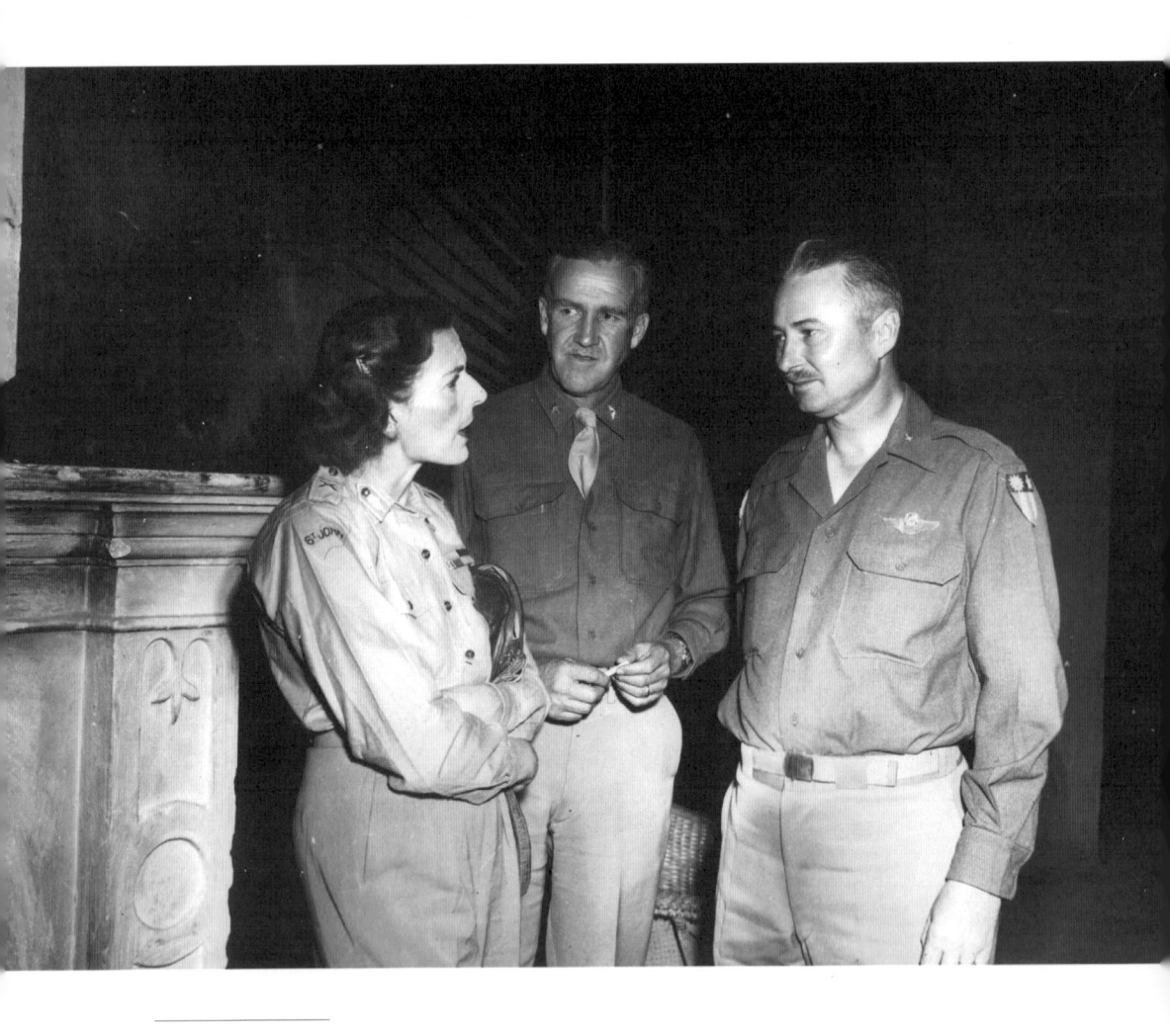

Lady Louis Mountbatten, Chief of Red Cross, and St. John's Ambulance Society of the Great Britain interacting in Bhamo, Burma.

路易斯・蒙巴頓總司令的夫人是英國紅十字會會長,她在造訪緬甸八莫時與聖約翰救護協會的成員交談。

Date of Photo 時間:May 3, 1945
Credits 來源:美國國家檔案館 Photo Courtesy of National Archives

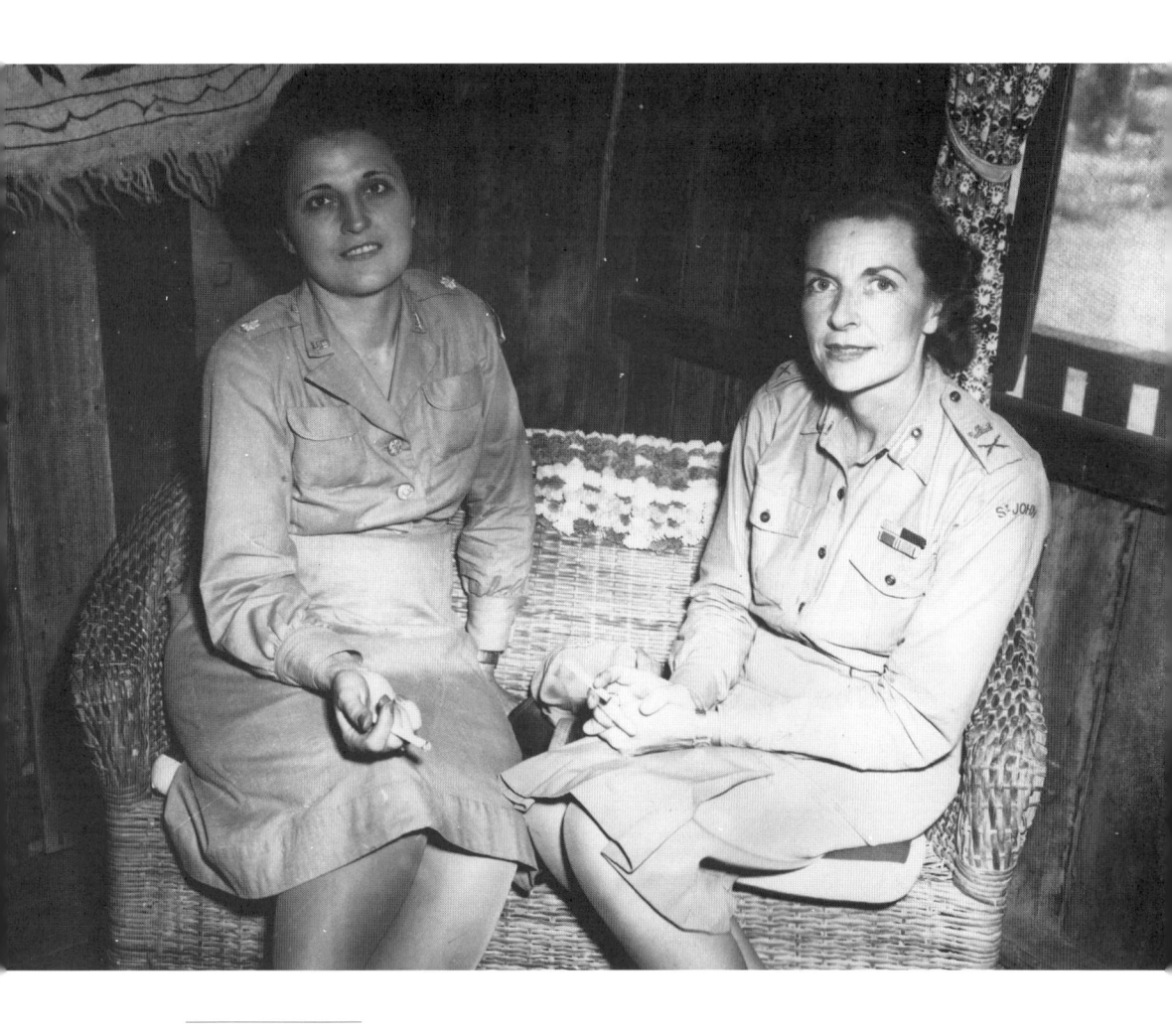

Lieutenant Colonel Agnes Mayle, Chief nurse of the India-Burma Theater, and Lady Louis Mountbatten, Chief of the Red Cross.

印度-緬甸戰區護理主任艾格尼絲・梅爾中校會晤路易斯・蒙巴頓總司令的夫人，夫人同時也是英國紅十字會會長。

Date of Photo 時間：May 2, 1945
Credits 來源：美國國家檔案館 Photo Courtesy of National Archives

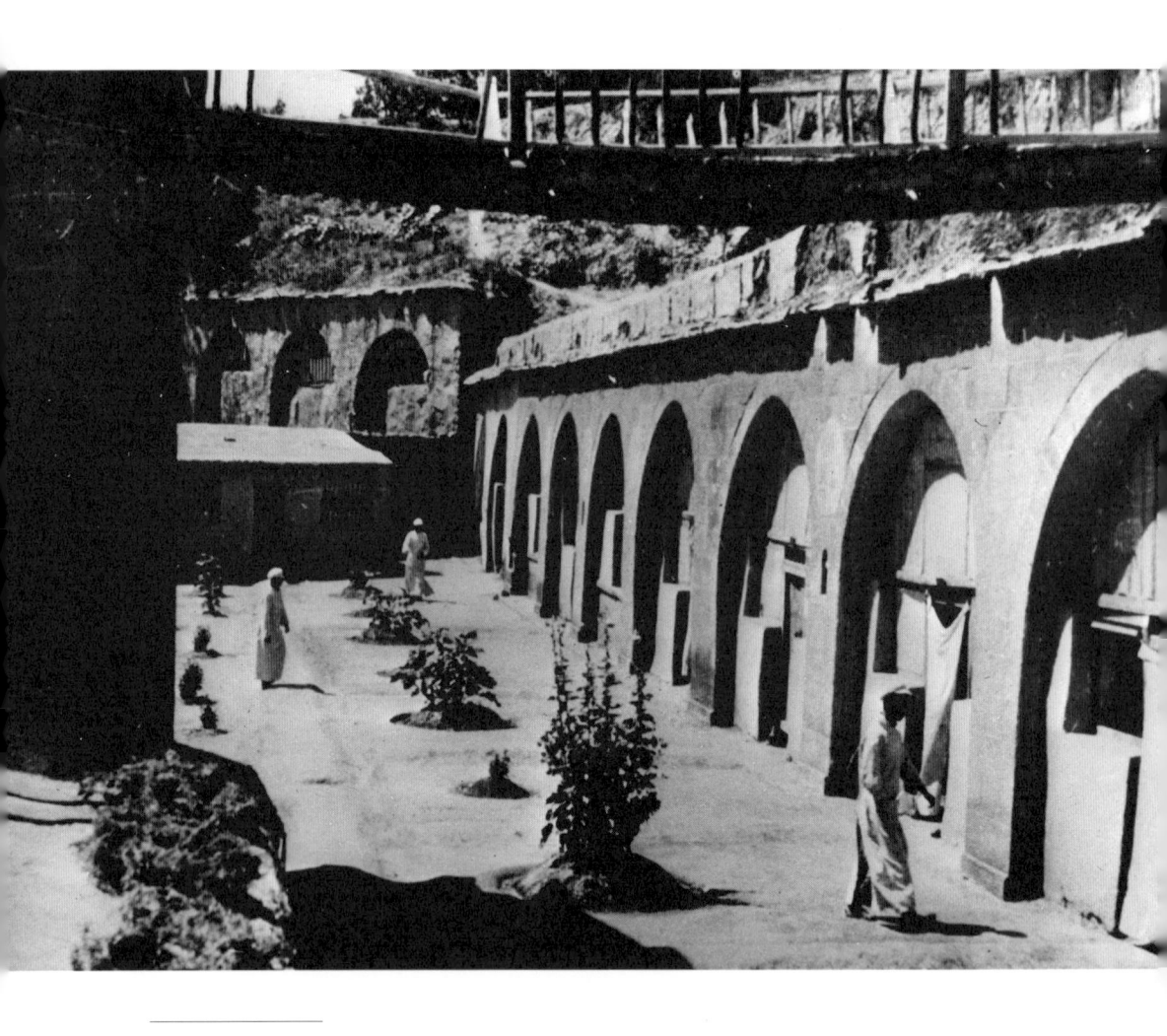

The surgical ward of the International Peace Hospital, China.
中國國際和平醫院的外科病房。

Date of Photo 時間：不詳 N/A
Credits 來源：美國國家檔案館 Photo Courtesy of National Archives

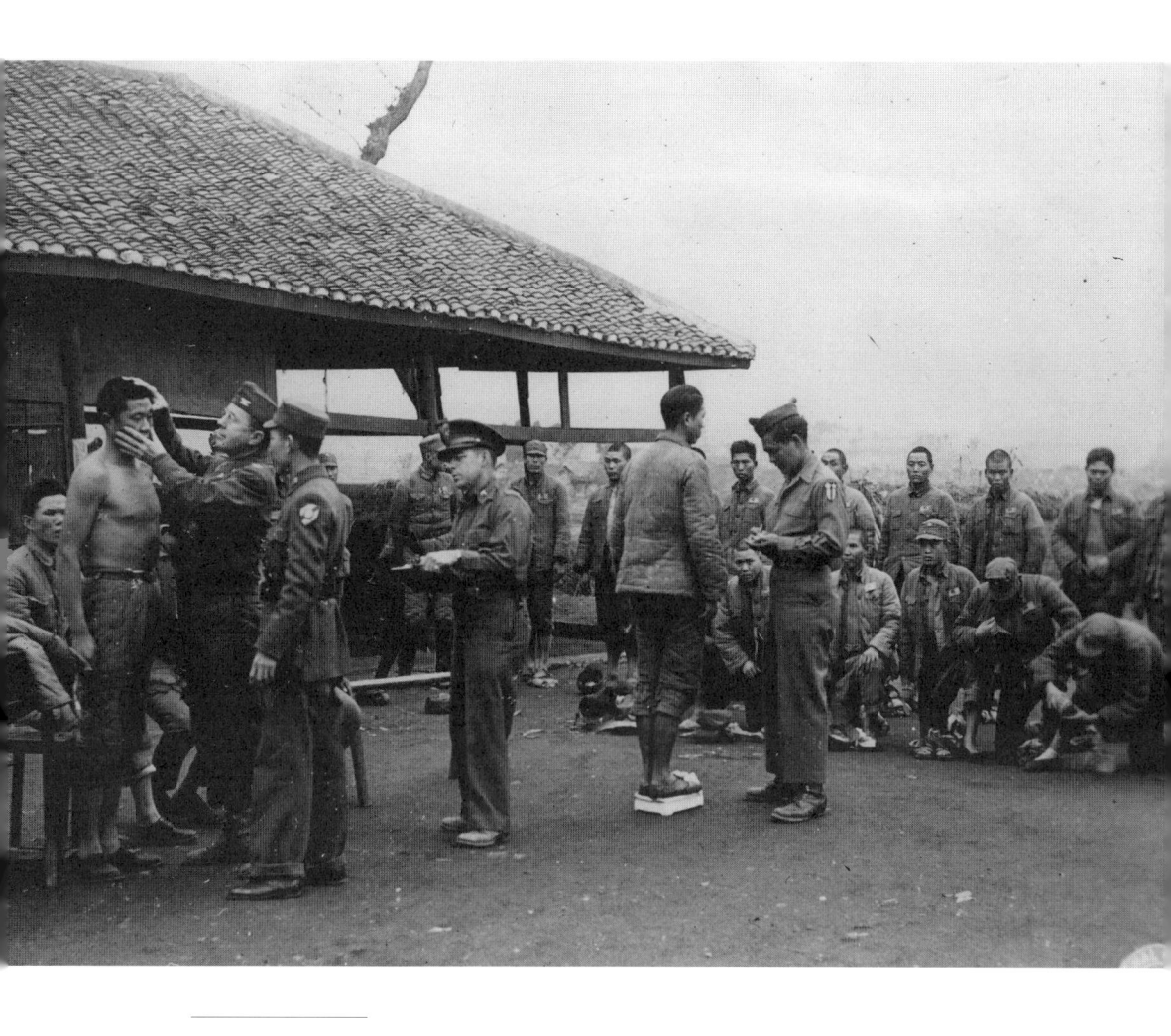

Director of the Nutrition Division of the Preventive Medicine Service of the Office of the U.S. Surgeon General, examined soldiers in Southwest China.

美國公共衛生局轄下預防醫學服務部門負責營養業務的主管在中國西南的一個基地為士兵看診。

Date of Photo 時間：March 15, 1945
Credits 來源：美國國家檔案館 Photo Courtesy of National Archives

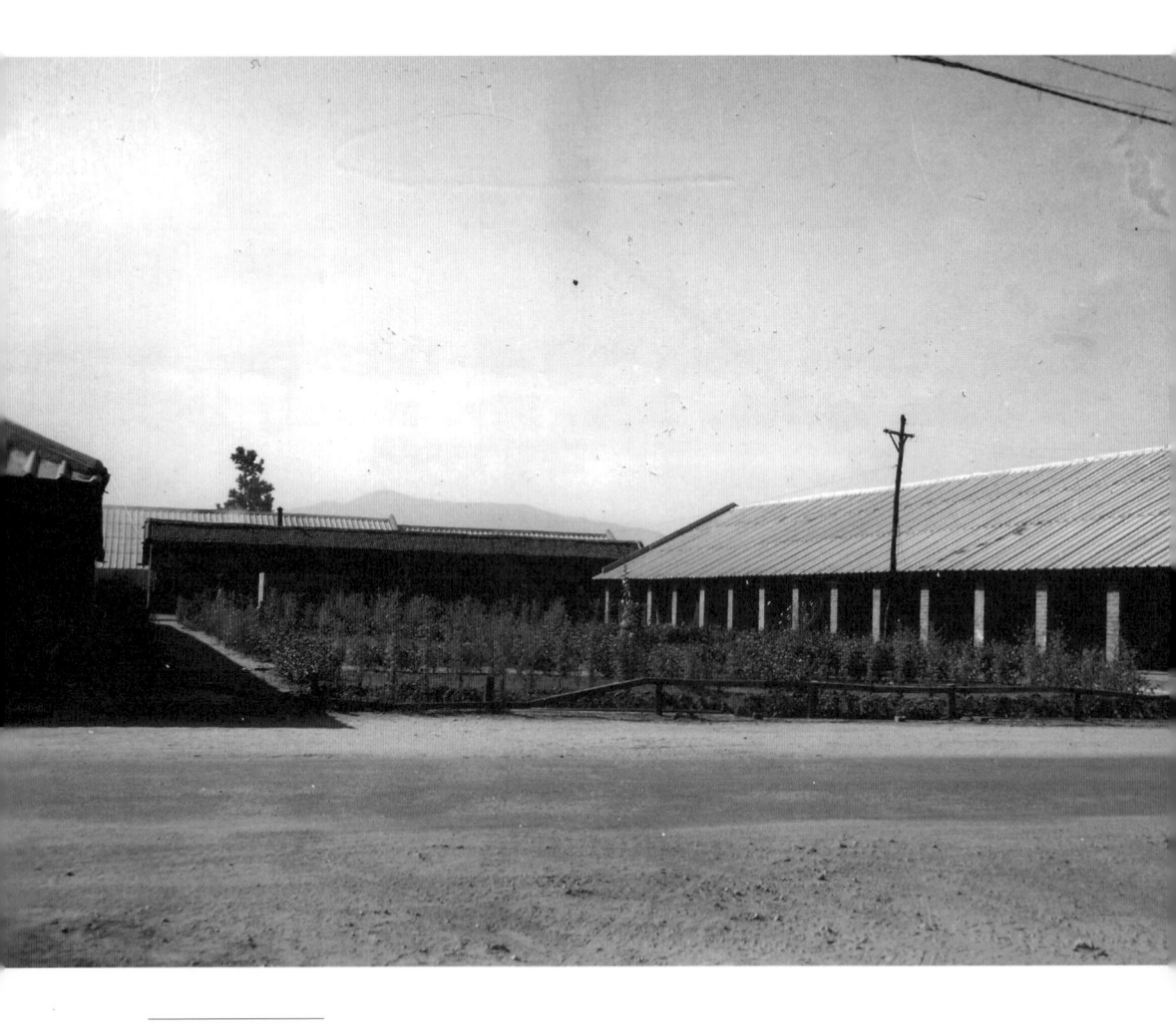

The United States 371st Station Hospital at the Ramgarh Training Center, India.

美軍第 371 駐紮地醫院,位於印度蘭姆伽的訓練中心。

Date of Photo 時間:July 16, 1948
Credits 來源:美國國家檔案館 Photo Courtesy of National Archives

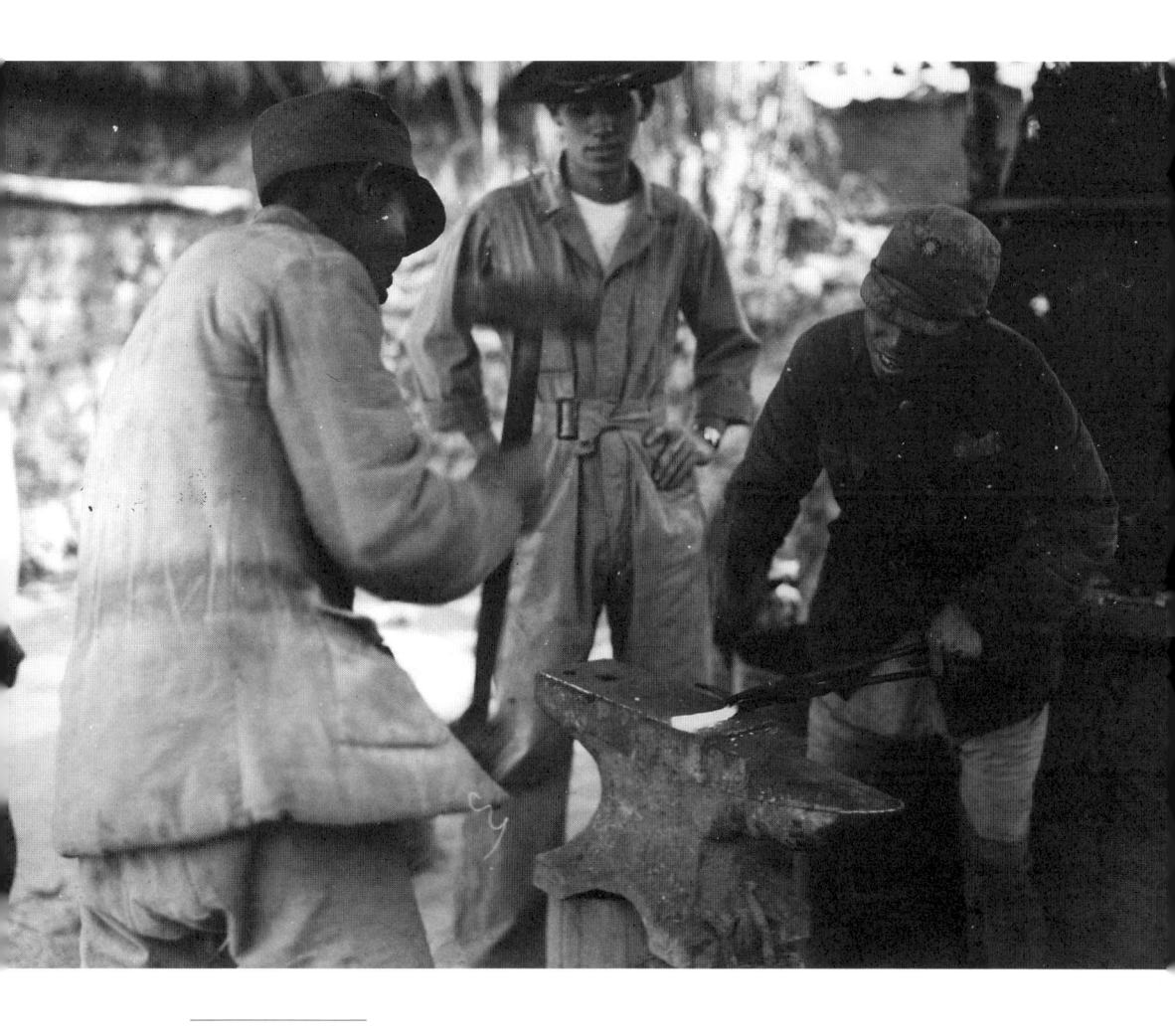

An American officer watching Chinese soldiers pounding old truck frames into horseshoes.

一名美國軍官看著中國士兵將舊卡車車架改造成馬蹄鐵。

Date of Photo 時間：May 12, 1945
Credits 來源：美國國家檔案館 Photo Courtesy of National Archives

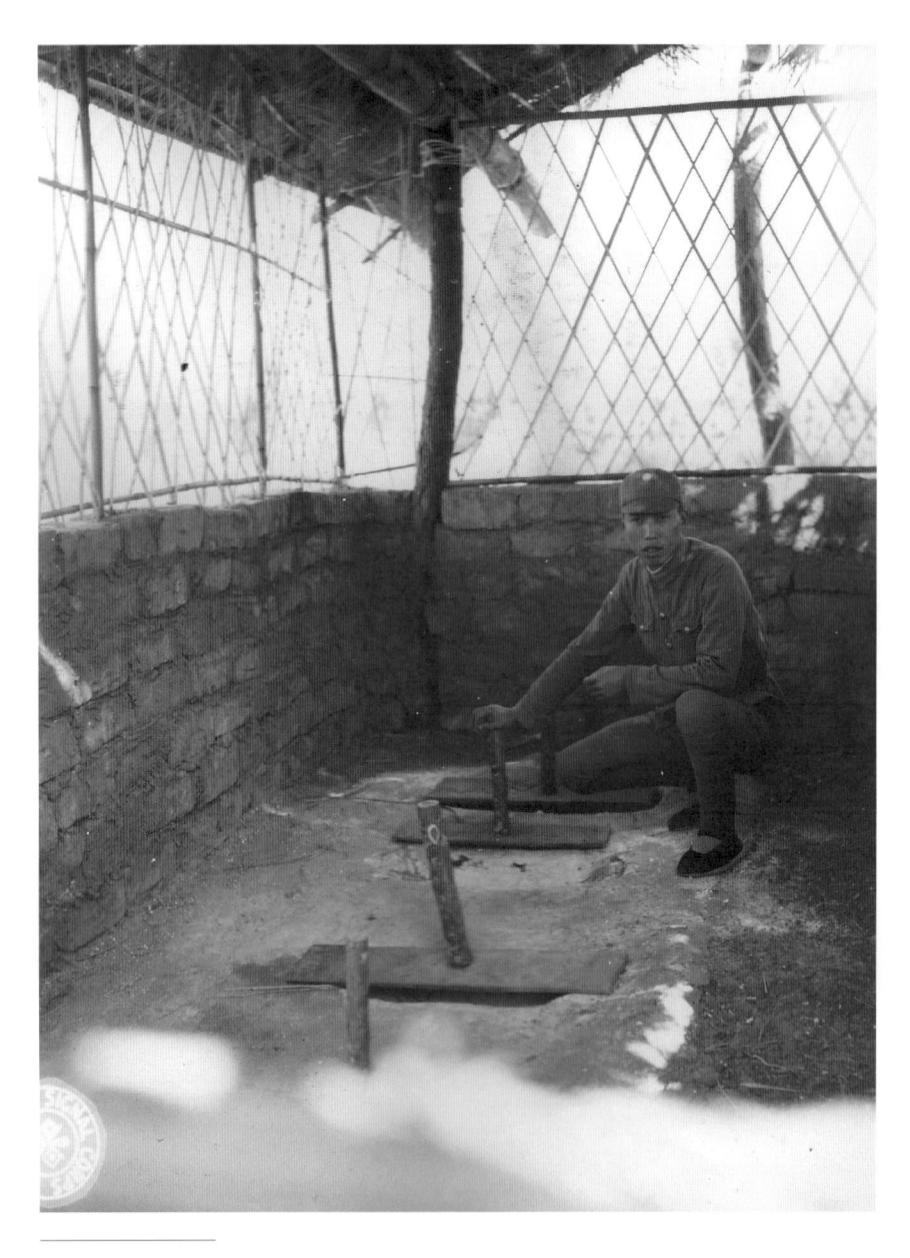

Model latrine used by Chinese personnel at 8th army 3RD Field Hospital.

國軍第八軍第三野戰醫院使用的茅廁。

Date of Photo 時間：July 16, 1948
Credits 來源：美國國家檔案館 Photo Courtesy of National Archives

A Chinese medic putting clothes into steam vat to delouse them. Clothes were steamed while Chinese soldiers took baths and sulfur treatment. When they were finished steaming, clothes were dried to be ready to wear.

中國醫護人員將衣物放入蒸汽槽中進行除虱處理。這是第八軍第三野戰醫院除虱過程的第三步。在中國士兵洗澡並接受硫磺治療的同時,也會以蒸汽處理他們的衣物。蒸汽處理結束後,將衣物晾乾後讓士兵穿上。

Date of Photo 時間:January, 1946
Credits 來源:美國國家檔案館 Photo Courtesy of National Archives

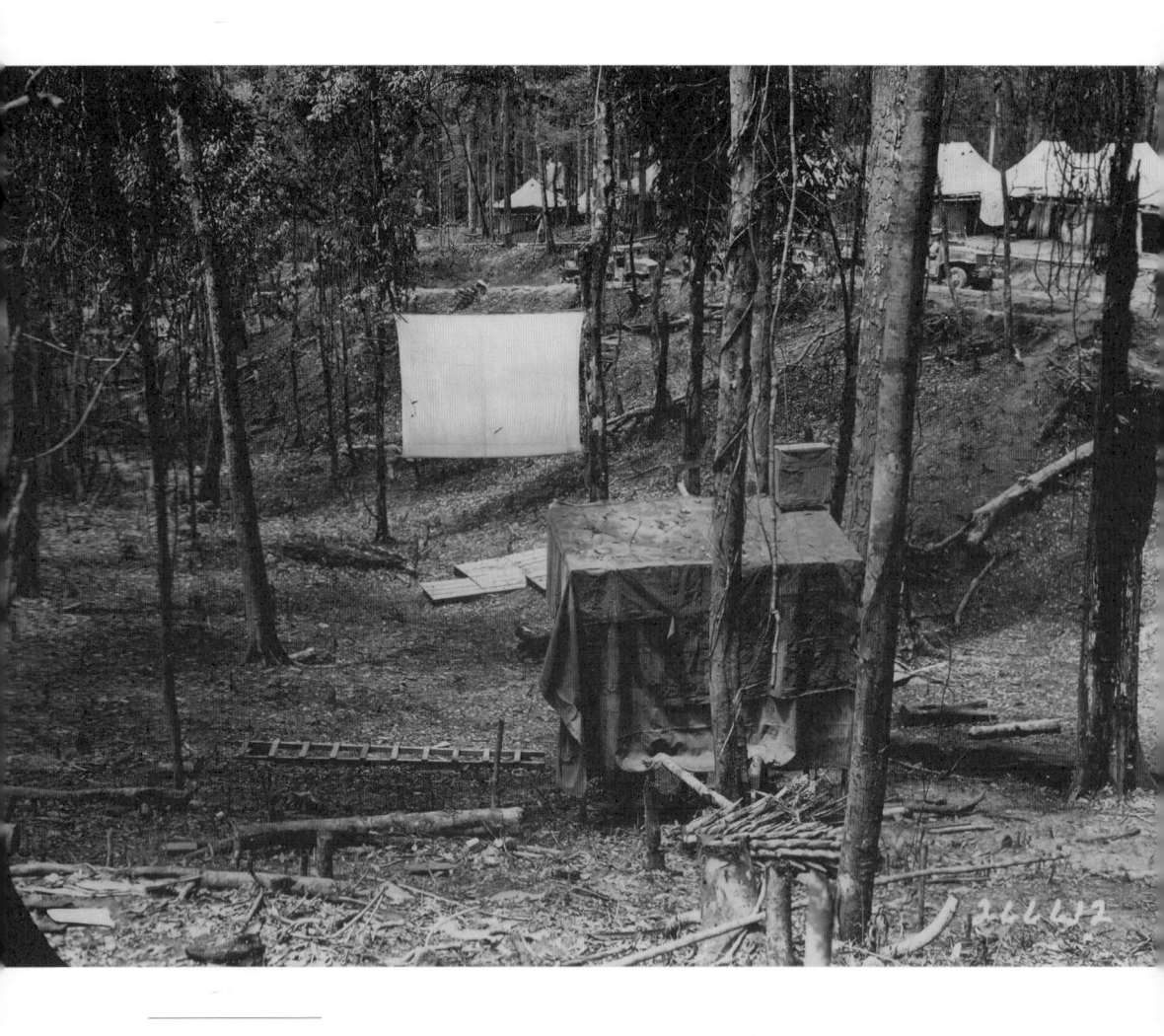

The amphitheater in the area of the 73rd Evacuation Hospital, Northern Burma.

第 73 後送醫院院區的手術室，位於緬甸北部。

Date of Photo 時間：May 22, 1945
Credits 來源：美國國家檔案館 Photo Courtesy of National Archives

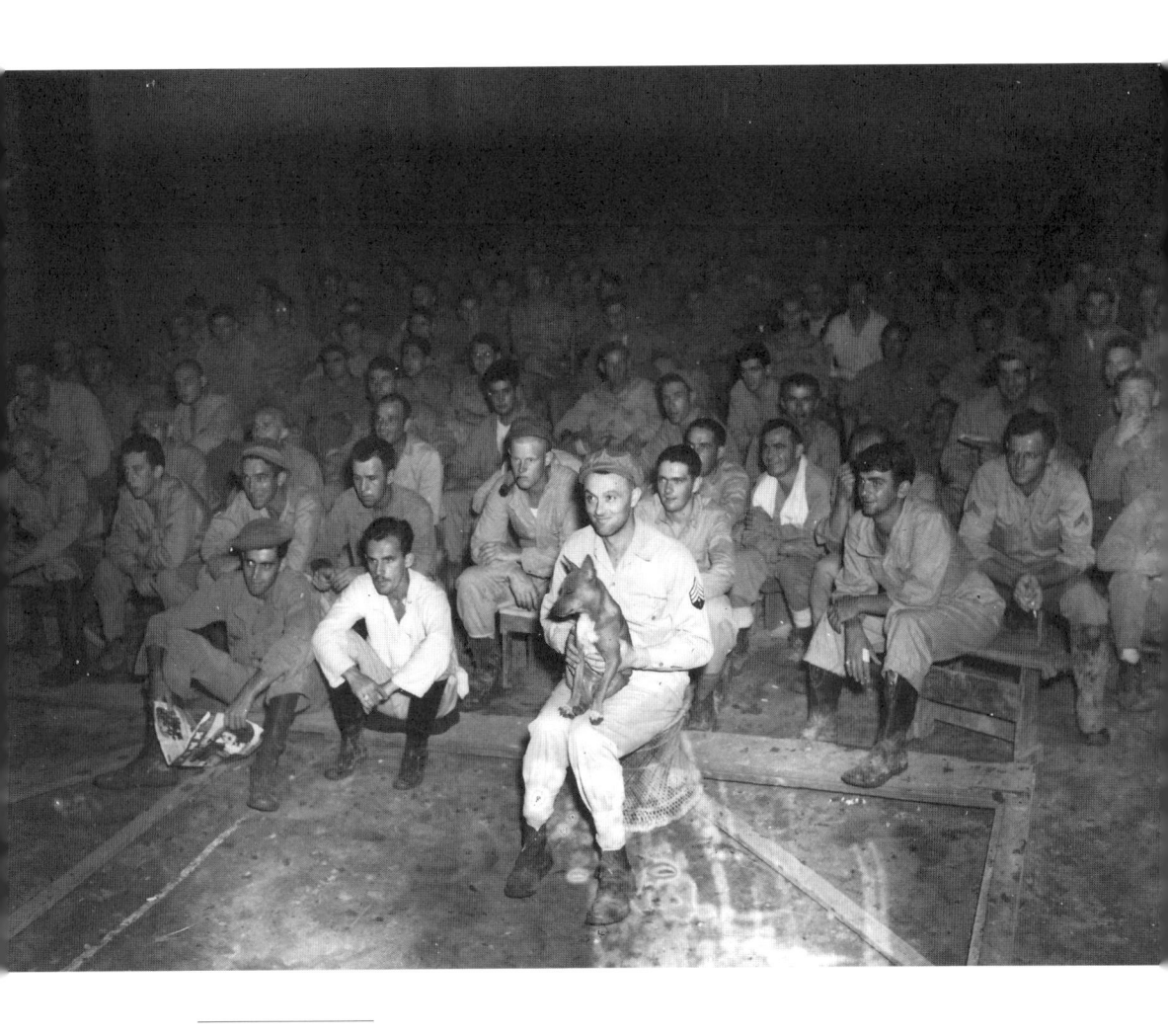

At the "Bamboo Bowl" Theater, officers, enlisted men, nurses, Chinese patients, and personnel from nearby camps would all sit to watch shows.

在別號「竹碗」的手術室裡,軍官、士兵、護士、中國病人和附近營地的軍人們都在等待演出開始。

Date of Photo 時間:September 1, 1948
Credits 來源:美國國家檔案館 Photo Courtesy of National Archives

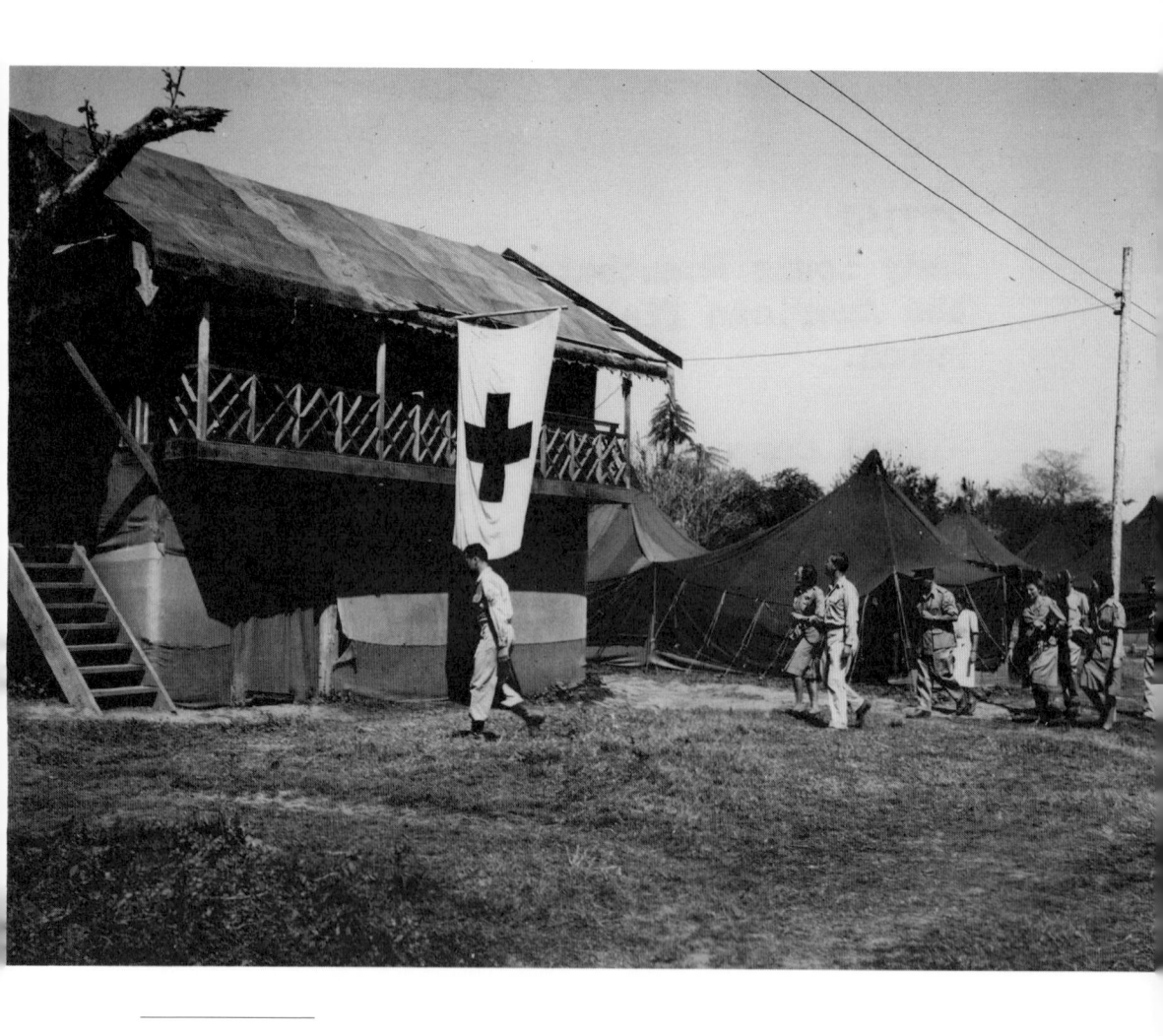

Lady Louis Mountbatten inspecting the American field hospital in Burma.

盟軍東南亞戰區總司令路易斯・蒙巴頓將軍的夫人正在視察位於緬甸的美國野戰醫院。

Date of Photo 時間：May 2, 1945
Credits 來源：美國國家檔案館 Photo Courtesy of National Archives

CONCLUSION

During World War II, the International Medical Relief Corps (IMRC) played a critical role in sustaining China's military and civilian populations. Amid war, famine, and disease, the IMRC and allied medical organizations provided essential care, training, and resources. Their efforts not only saved lives but also laid the foundation for China's modern healthcare system.

One of the most significant advancements in wartime medical care was the use of air transport, particularly C-47 aircraft, which revolutionized medical evacuation and supply distribution. Wounded soldiers could now be transported from the front lines to field hospitals far more quickly, drastically improving survival rates. In remote regions where aircraft could not reach, injured troops relied on oxen to carry them across rugged terrain to waiting medical teams. But despite these relentless logistical challenges, medical personnel were determined to adapt.

In order to further push forward the IMRC's humanitarian activities, elevations in medical technology, such as blood transfusion technology were relayed. Although many in China associated blood loss with a weakening of vitality, making voluntary donations rare, medical teams combated this resistance by launching public campaigns emphasizing nationalism and altruism, while also offering food incentives to increase donor turnout. These efforts gradually stabilized blood supplies, ensuring life-saving transfusions for wounded soldiers.

However, political tensions within China often threatened these operations and proper communication. Deep-seated distrust between the Guomindang and the Chinese Communist Party, along with corruption and bureaucratic inefficiencies, frequently disrupted supply chains and medical coordination. Yet, in the face of these setbacks, American and Chinese personnel worked together to establish field hospitals and medical training programs that proved vital to not only China's war effort against the Imperial Japanese Army but also all of the Allied Powers. Through initiatives like the Emergency Medical Service Training School and the American Bureau for Medical Advancement in China, more than 13,000 Chinese medical workers were trained in battlefield medicine, emergency care, and public health—investments that would have lasting effects beyond the war.

And, despite the medical advancements, wartime conditions remained grueling.

In the China-Burma-India Theater, hospitals operated under extreme scarcity. Makeshift surgical units were often housed in tents, staffed by small teams who performed operations with minimal equipment and supplies. Doctors and nurses were forced to improvise, using limited stocks of sulfa drugs, iodine, and alcohol for disinfection. In some cases, old bandages were washed and reused, heightening the risk of infection. Meanwhile, shortages of protective gear left medical personnel vulnerable to diseases like typhoid and tuberculosis. Exhausted and often malnourished, they worked through relentless conditions, treating hundreds of patients per day with little rest.

Beyond physical injuries, the psychological toll of war was severe. Chinese soldiers and civilians alike suffered from trauma, yet psychiatric care remained scarce. While Western medical missionaries had introduced psychiatric treatment in China in the late 19th century, mental health remained a low priority during the war. Existing institutions, such as the Canton Hospital for the Insane and Shanghai Mercy Hospital, provided limited services, but these were largely inaccessible to the broader population. The war's devastation underscored the need for better psychiatric care, laying the groundwork for gradual improvements in the decades that followed.

Despite many more immense challenges, the IMRC's contributions ultimately had an uplifting lasting impact. Their ability to operate under extreme conditions, develop innovative medical solutions, and train a new generation of healthcare workers helped shape China's post-war medical landscape. While the war exposed the weaknesses of China's healthcare system, it also spurred advancements in medical training, public health initiatives, and emergency response strategies.

In the face of overwhelming adversity, medical personnel from China and the United States demonstrated extraordinary commitment to saving lives. The IMRC's efforts spanned beyond World War II but also set a precedent for modern medical relief efforts. Their story remains a testament to the vital role of medical professionals in times of crisis, the enduring impact of humanitarian aid, and collaboration between vastly differing nations.

結語

第二次世界大戰期間，國際醫療救護隊致力於維持中國軍民的生命安全，發揮了關鍵作用。面對戰爭、飢荒與疾病，國際醫療救護隊及其他盟軍醫療組織提供了不可或缺的醫療照護、專業訓練與物資支援。他們的努力不僅挽救了無數生命，更為中國現代醫療體系奠定了基礎。

　　戰時醫療最重要的進步之一，是空運技術的運用，尤其是 C-47 運輸機，大幅革新了傷兵後送與醫療物資的補給方式。傷員得以從前線迅速轉送至戰地醫院，顯著提高了存活率。在飛機無法抵達的偏遠地區，傷兵則仰賴牛車翻山越嶺，將他們送往待命中的醫療隊。即便後勤工作困難重重，醫護人員依然堅持克服種種障礙，因地制宜地展開救治。

　　為了進一步推動國際醫療救護隊的人道救援行動，當時醫療科技的發展亦有所突破，例如輸血的普及。儘管當時中國社會普遍認為失血會削弱人體元氣，導致捐血意願低落，醫療隊透過宣傳民族主義與互助精神，加上提供食物作為獎勵，有效提升了捐血率，逐漸穩定了戰地輸血所需。

　　然而，國內政治局勢動盪也對醫療行動與溝通協調造成了重大威脅。國民政府與中國共產黨之間的互相猜忌、政治腐敗與貪官污吏，屢次阻礙物資供應與醫療協調。儘管如此，中美醫療人員依然攜手合作，設立戰地醫院與醫護訓練計畫，對中國抗戰與盟軍戰事都至關重要。透過如戰時衛生人員訓練所與美國醫藥助華會等機構，超過 13,000 名中國醫護人員接受了戰地醫學、急救與公共衛生的訓練，這些行動對戰後中國的醫療發展產生了深遠影響。

　　即便醫療技術有所進步，戰地條件依舊艱苦。在中緬印戰區，醫院的物資極度匱乏，臨時手術站多設於帳篷內，僅靠少數醫護人員與簡陋器材應付大量手術。醫護人員時常必須隨機應變，僅以少量磺胺藥、碘酒與酒精消毒，有時甚至重複使用繃帶、用熱水替代消毒劑，導致感染風險極高。防護裝備的不足，也讓醫護人員暴露於傷寒、肺結核等傳染病之中。即使疲憊不堪、營養不良，醫護隊仍日夜救治數百名病患。

　　除身體創傷外，戰爭的心理創傷同樣嚴重。無論軍民，皆飽受戰爭帶來的精神壓力與創傷症候群之苦，但當時精神醫療資源極其稀少。雖然西方傳教士於 19 世紀晚期將精神醫學引進中國，但至抗戰時期，精神疾病並未被廣泛重視，現存的如廣州惠愛醫癲院與上海普慈療養院等機構，也無法滿足廣大需求。戰爭的破壞讓社會意識到心理醫療的重要性，為戰後心理醫學發展奠定了基礎。

儘管挑戰重重，美國醫藥助華會的貢獻最終產生了深遠且正面的影響。他們在極端環境下持續救治、研發創新的醫療方法與培育新一代醫護人員，深刻影響了戰後中國醫療體系的重建與發展。戰爭暴露了中國醫療制度的脆弱，但也促進了醫學教育、公共衛生與緊急醫療體系的現代化。

儘管面對種種艱難險阻，中美醫護人員展現了非凡的奉獻精神。美國醫藥助華會的行動不僅超越了二戰，更為近代國際醫療救援樹立了典範。他們的故事證明，危難之際醫護專業有多寶貴，人道救援也會帶來長遠影響，而且跨國合作充滿各種可能性，永遠值得被銘記與傳承。

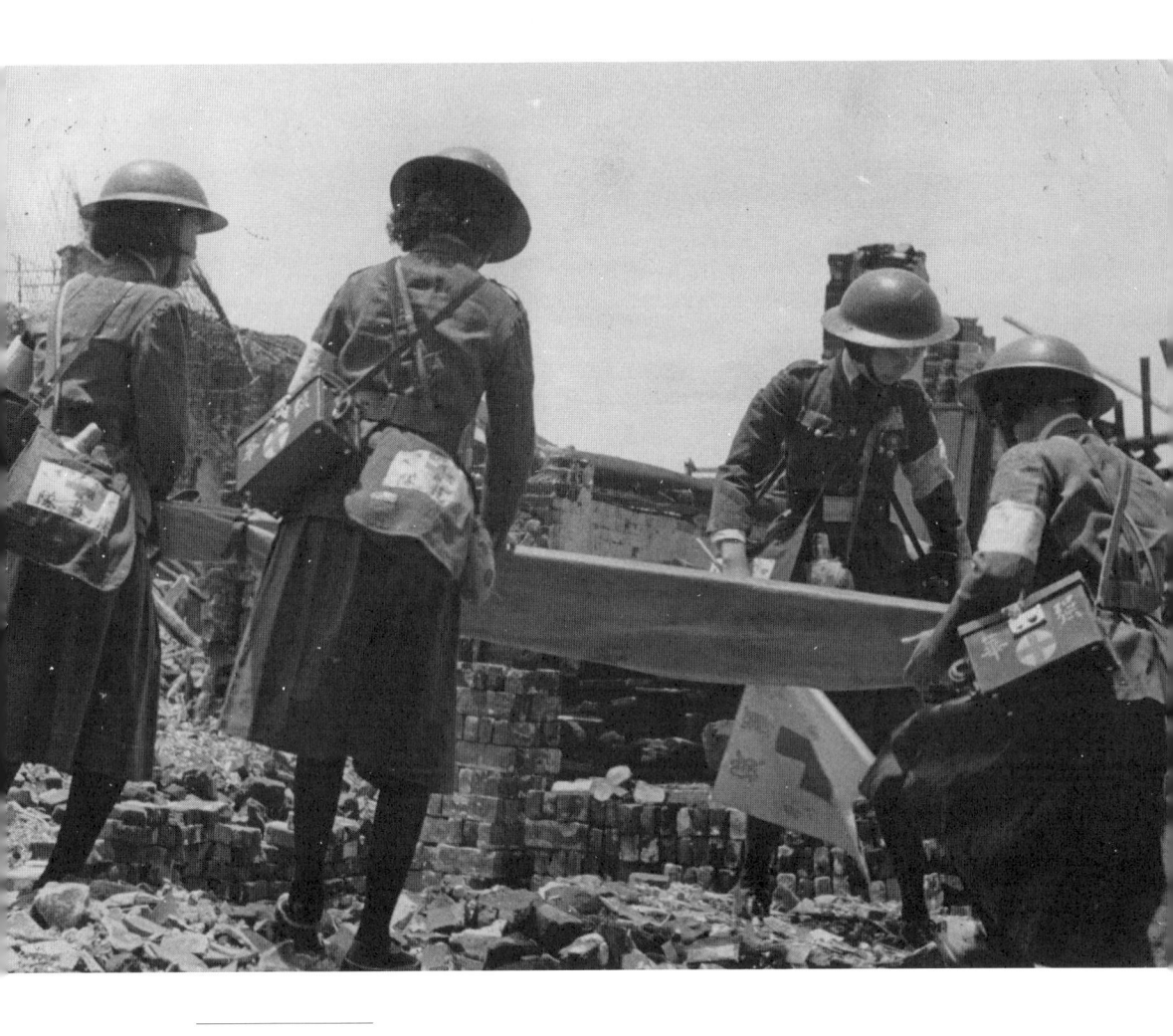

Teams of young emergency trained medical aids helped to set up and treat wounded soldiers on site.

受過緊急醫療訓練的年輕醫護隊伍在戰場協助搭建救護站並救治傷兵。

Date of Photo 時間：不詳 N/A
Credits 來源：美國國家檔案館 Photo Courtesy of National Archives

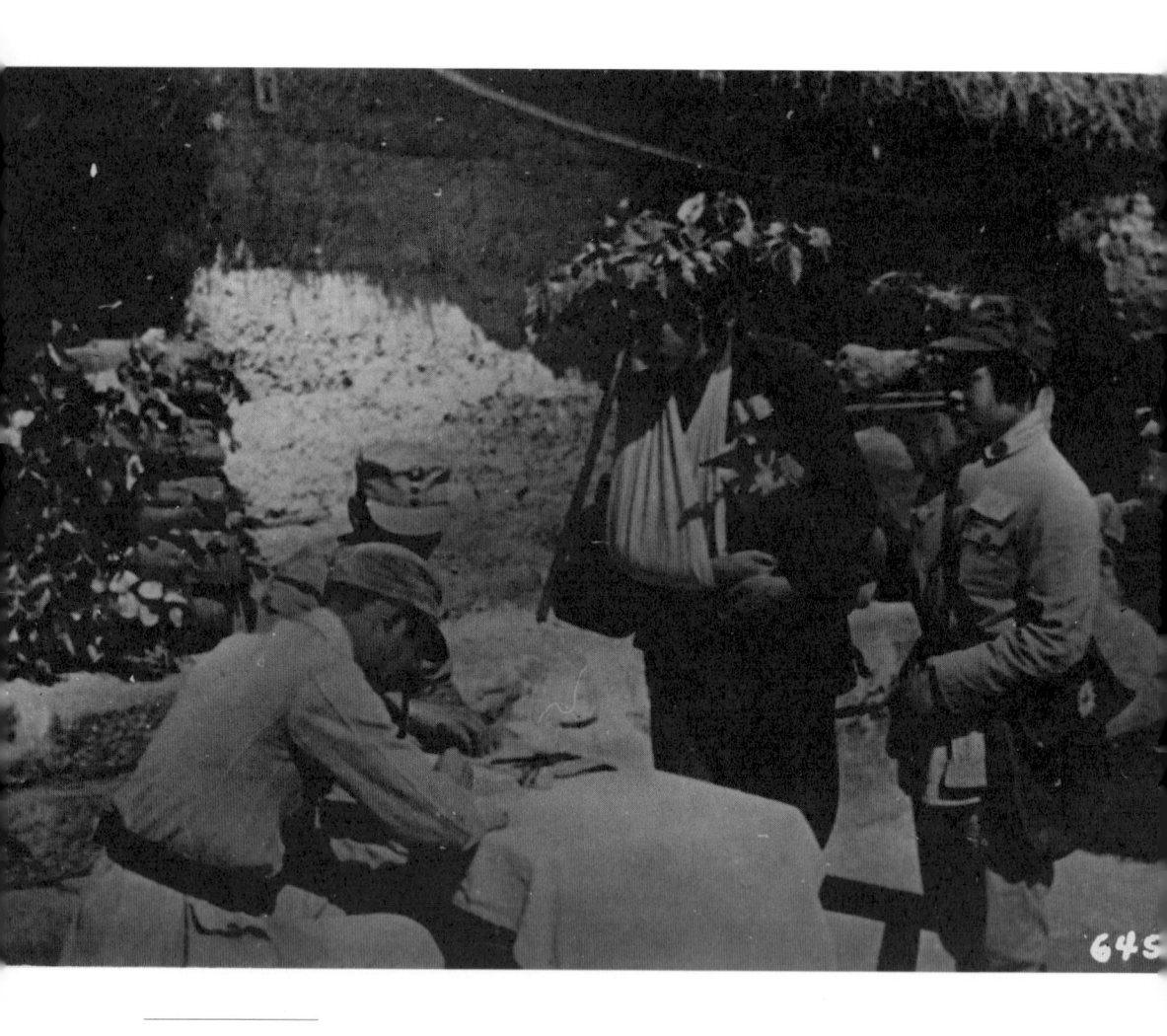

Wounded Chinese soldiers receive treatment and hospitalization on site, even whilst wearing their camouflage hats.

受傷的中國士兵即便仍戴著具有迷彩掩蔽裝飾的帽子,也在戰場上接受治療與收容。

Date of Photo 時間:不詳 N/A
Credits 來源:美國國家檔案館 Photo Courtesy of National Archives

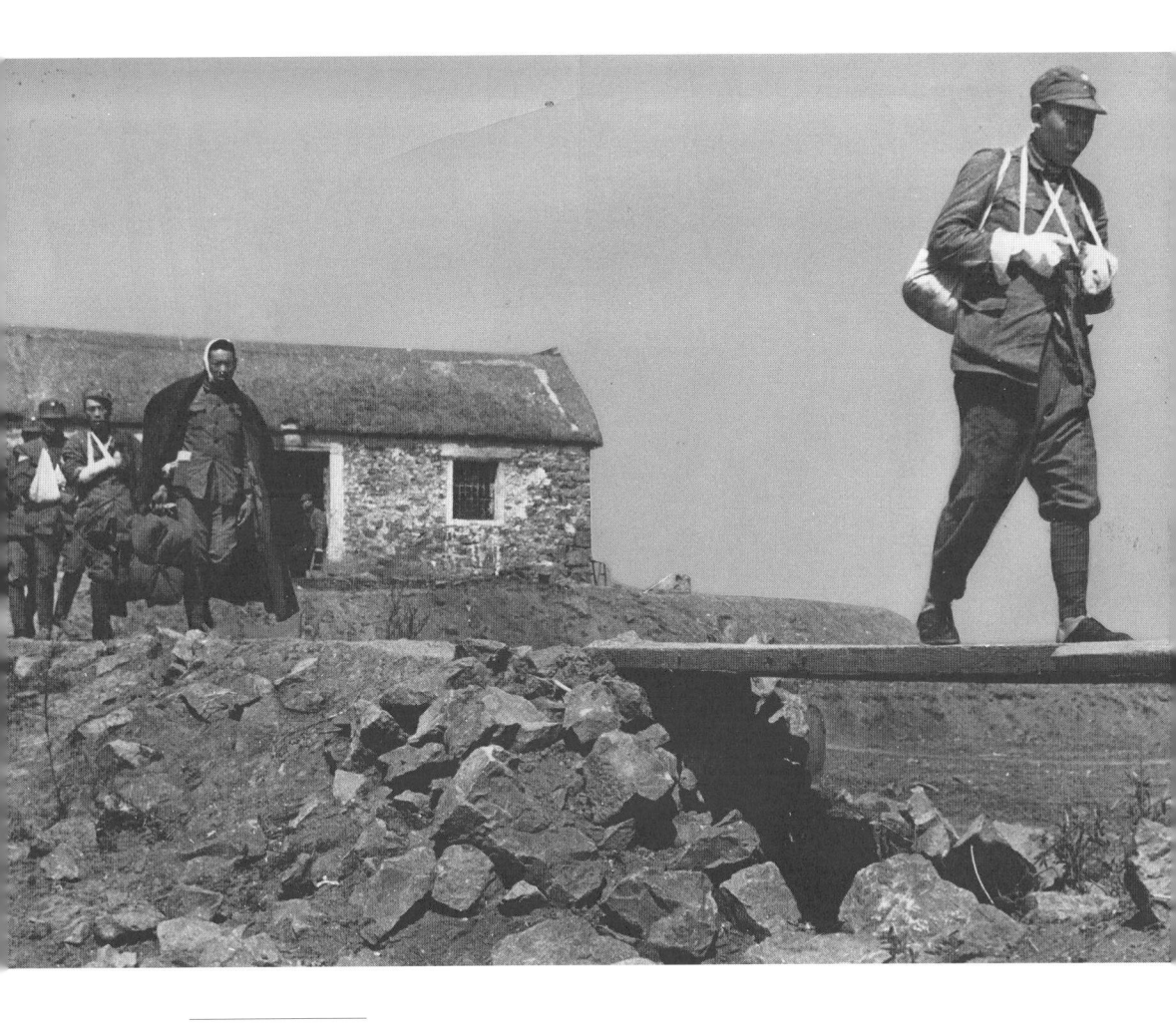

Chinese wounded in the battle of Taierchuang marched six miles to a railroad outside the city to be transported to hospitals outside the war zone.

台兒莊戰役期間,受傷的中國士兵徒步六英里至城外鐵路,隨後被轉送至戰區外的醫院救治。

Date of Photo 時間:March 25, 1943
Credits 來源:美國國家檔案館 Photo Courtesy of National Archives

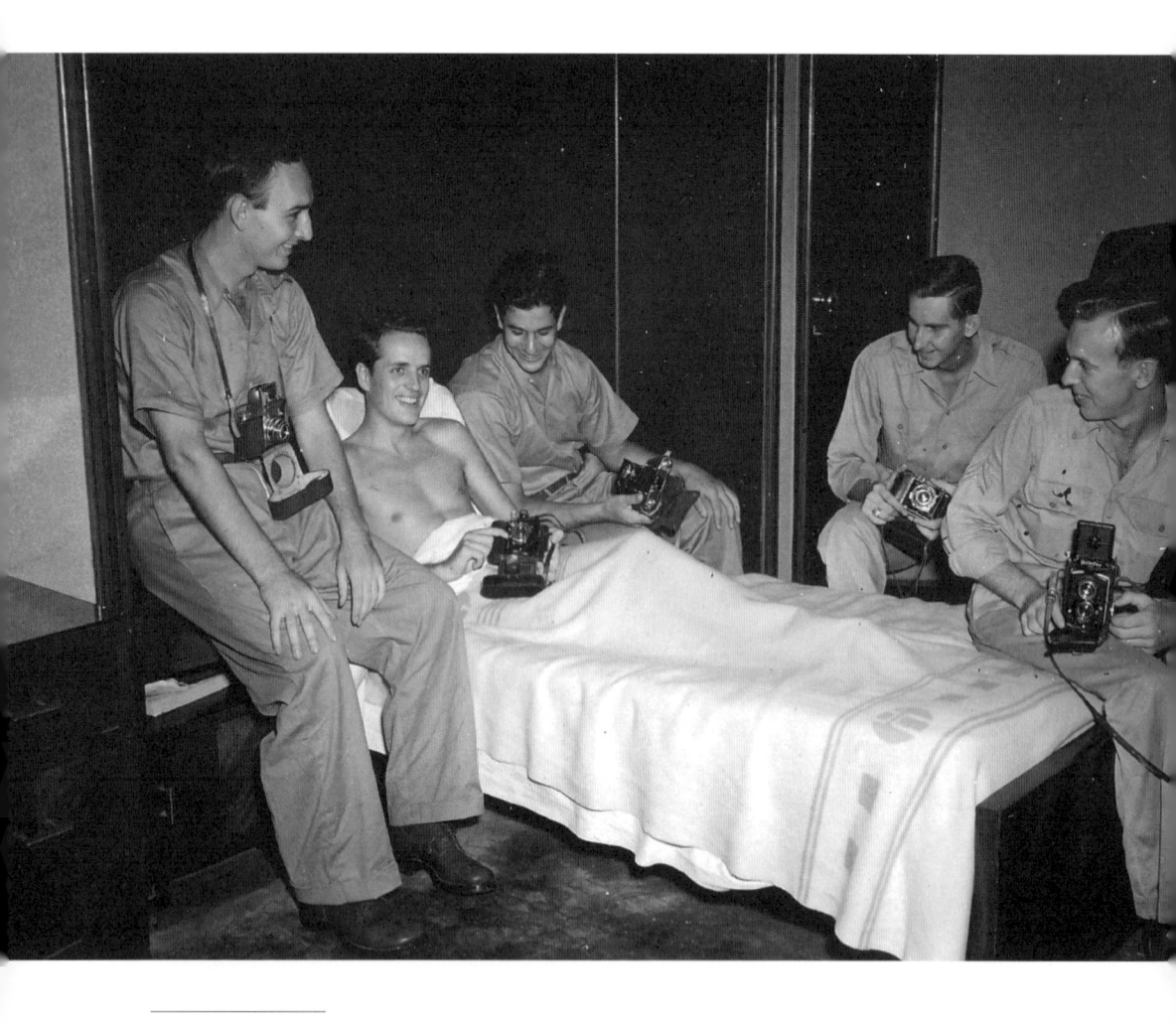

Liberation of American prisoners receiving treatment at St. Luke's Hospital in Shanghai, China.

獲救的美國戰俘在中國上海的同仁醫院中接受治療。

Date of Photo 時間：October 9, 1945
Credits 來源：美國國家檔案館 Photo Courtesy of National Archives

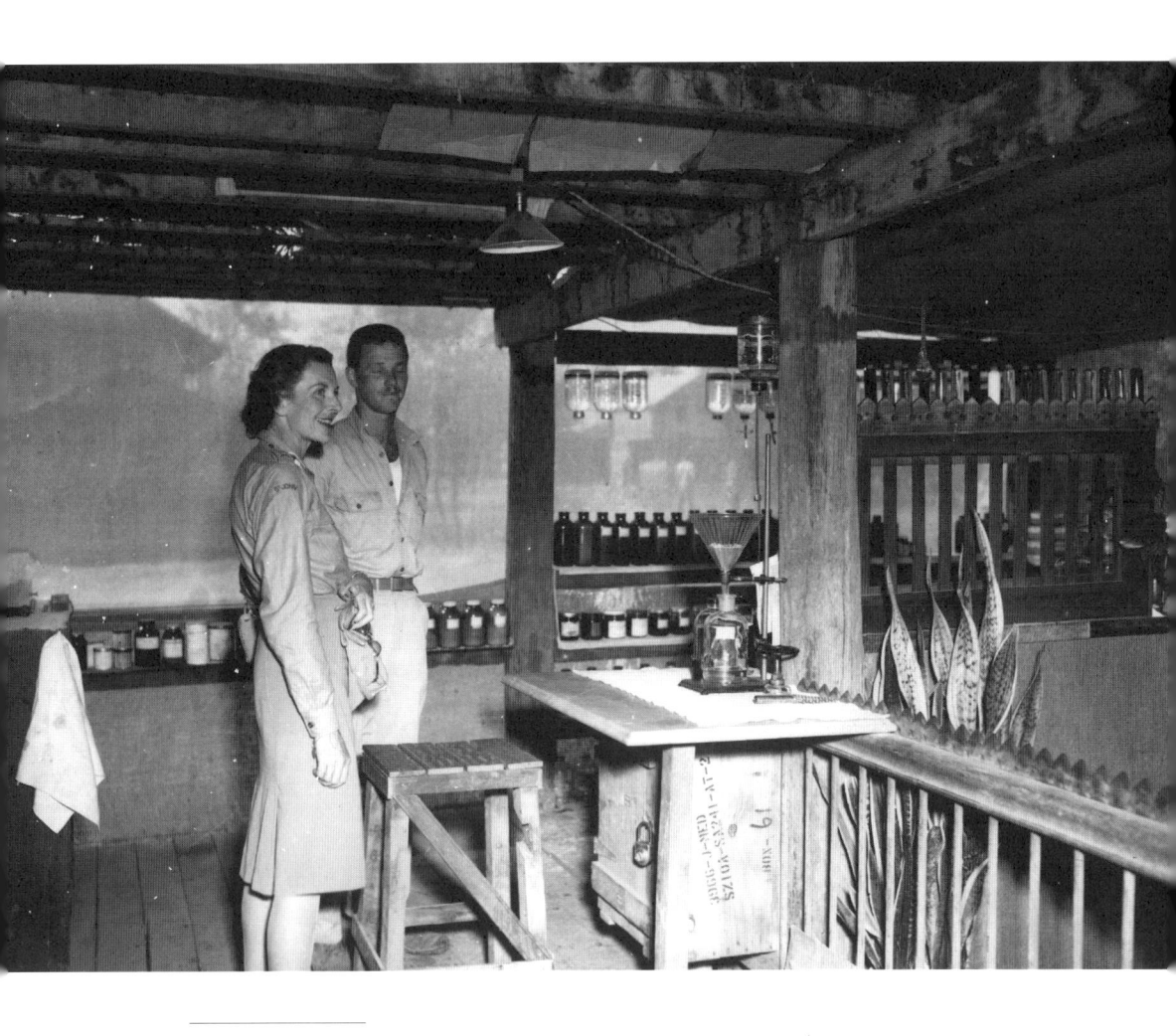

Lady Louis Mountbatten, wife of the Supreme commander of the Allied Forces in the southeast of Asia, visited the 44th Field Hospital during her visit to Bhamo, Burma.

盟軍東南亞戰區總司令路易斯・蒙巴頓將軍的夫人在造訪緬甸八莫期間,前往第 44 野戰醫院慰問。

Date of Photo 時間:March 6, 1945
Credits 來源:美國國家檔案館 Photo Courtesy of National Archives

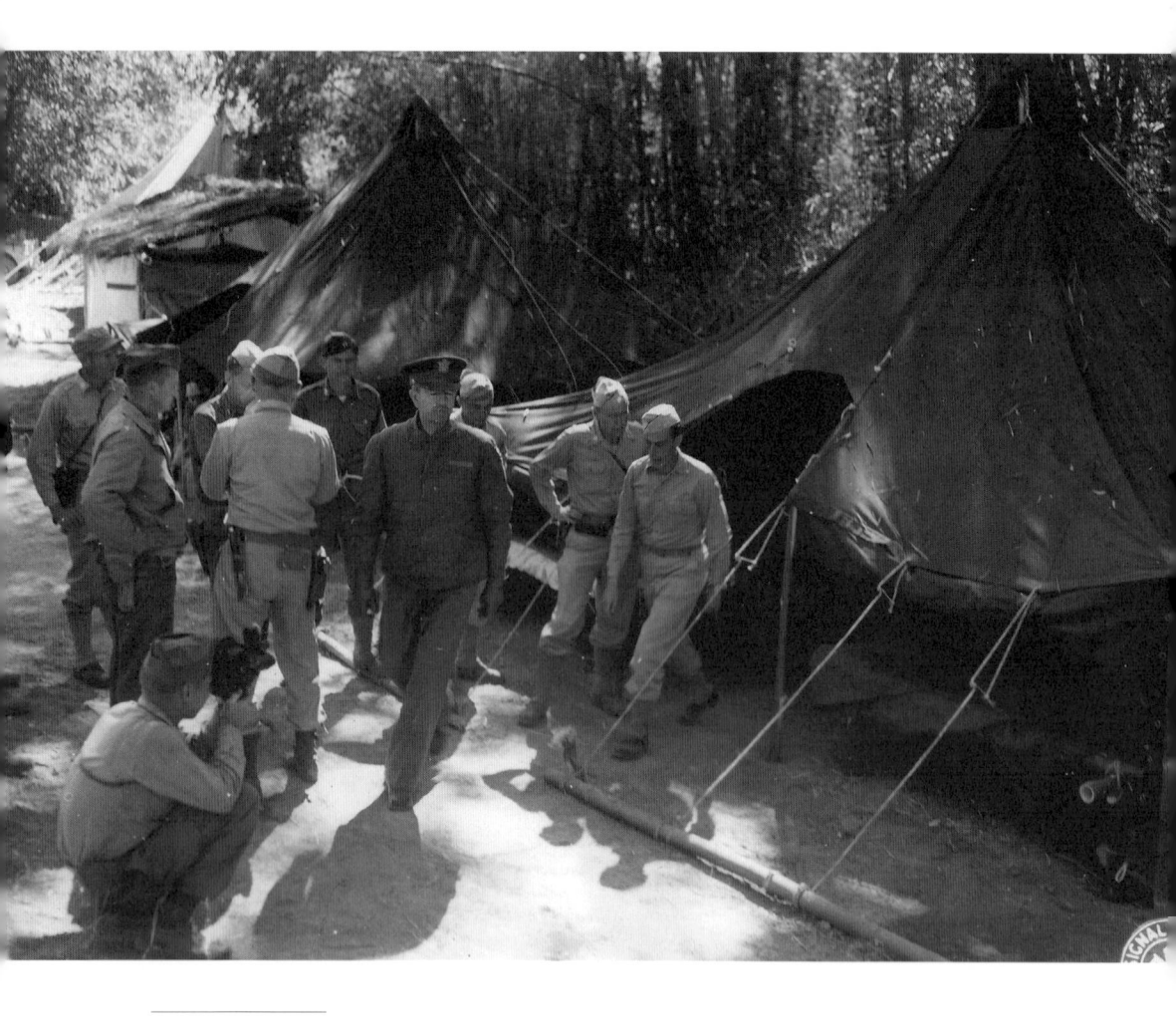

Major General Albert C. Wedemeyer standing near a portable surgical hospital near the Burma border.

魏德邁將軍在緬甸邊境附近的前線視察移動式外科醫院。

Date of Photo 時間：不詳 N/A
Credits 來源：美國國家檔案館 Photo Courtesy of National Archives

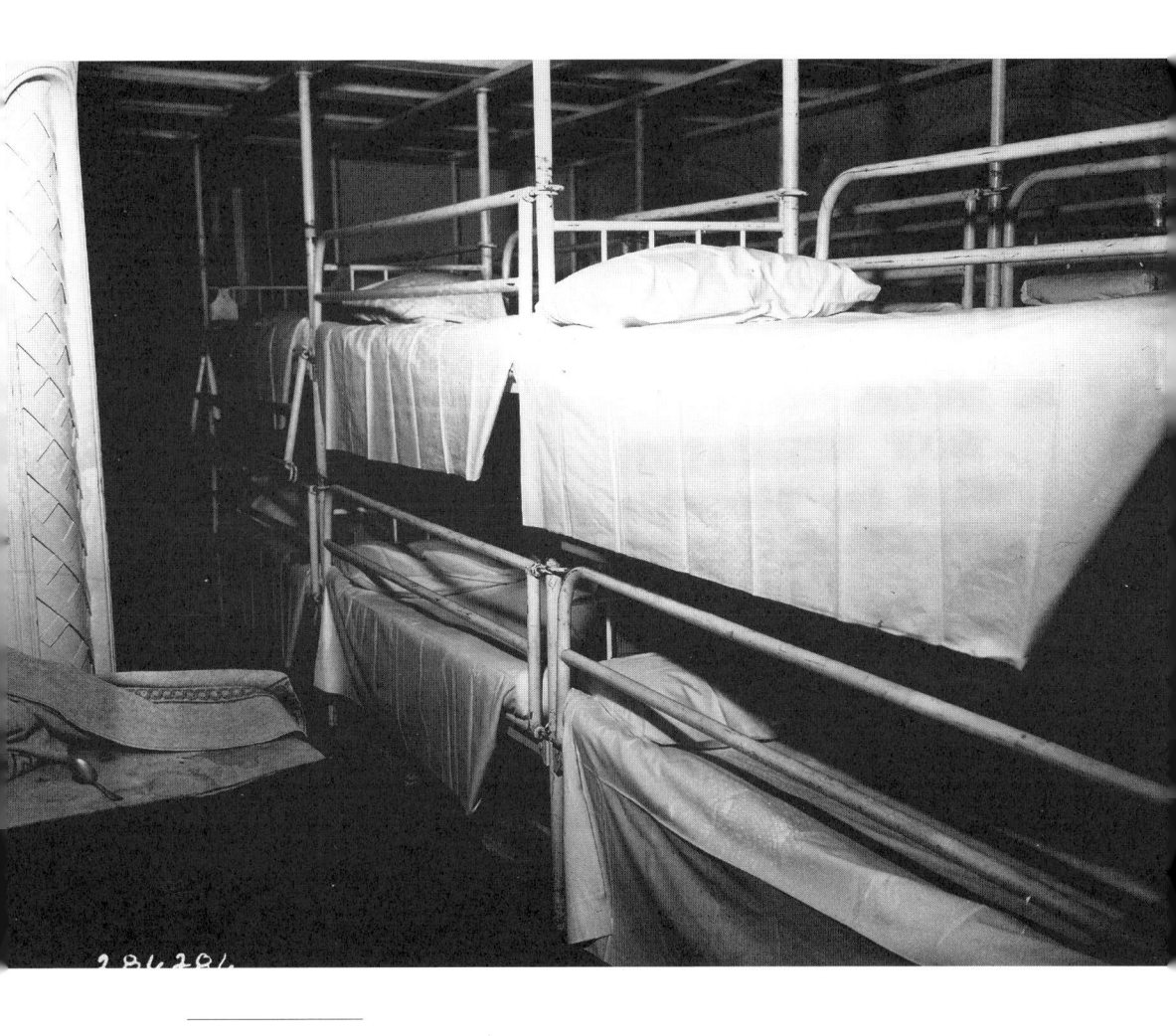

A picture of the sick bay of a transport, taken at the San Francisco Port of Embarkation.

一艘運輸船上的醫務室,攝於舊金山登船港。

Date of Photo 時間:1942
Credits 來源:美國國家檔案館 Photo Courtesy of National Archives

参考資料
References

Introduction and Conclusion

1. "Hospital Units in the China-Burma-India Theater of World War II." 2025. Cbi-Theater.com. 2025. https://cbi-theater.com/hospitals/_cbi_hospitals.html.
2. "United China Relief – Museum of Chinese in America." n.d. Www.mocanyc.org. https://www.mocanyc.org/collections/stories/united-china-relief/.
3. "WWII Campaigns: China Defensive." n.d. Www.history.army.mil. https://www.history.army.mil/brochures/72-38/72-38.htm.
4. Back, George I., and George Raynor Thompson. 2019. "Military Communication - World War II and after | Britannica." In Encyclopædia Britannica. https://www.britannica.com/technology/military-communication/World-War-II-and-after. Wikipedia Contributors. 2024. "Radioteletype." Wikipedia. Wikimedia Foundation. October 27, 2024.
5. Firsov, Fridrikh I., Harvey Klehr, John Earl Haynes, and Lynn Visson. Secret Cables of the Comintern, 1933-1943. Yale University Press, 2014. http://www.jstor.org/stable/j.ctt13x1tgv.

Infrastructure, Transportation, and Communications

1. Mamlok, Robert. 2018. *The International Medical Relief Corps in Wartime China, 1937-1945*. McFarland.
2. Mamlok, Robert. 2018. *The International Medical Relief Corps in Wartime China, 1937-1945*. McFarland.
3. Rampersad, Krystal, and Michael Montalbano. 2024. "A Life on the Frontlines: The Legacy of Norman Bethune (1890–1939)." Cureus, August. https://doi.org/10.7759/cureus.67286.
4. The Editors of *Encyclopedia Britannica*. 2017. "Second Sino-Japanese War | Summary, Facts, & Results." In Encyclopædia Britannica. https://www.britannica.com/event/Second-Sino-Japanese-War.
5. Wikipedia Contributors. 2019. "China–United States Relations." Wikipedia. Wikimedia Foundation. April 8, 2019. https://en.wikipedia.org/wiki/China%E2%80%93United_States_relations.
6. Wikipedia Contributors. 2019. "Republic of China (1912-1949)." Wikipedia. Wikimedia Foundation. November 3, 2019. https://en.wikipedia.org/wiki/Republic_of_China_(1912%E2%80%931949).
7. Wikipedia Contributors. 2025. "Dwarkanath Kotnis." Wikipedia. Wikimedia Foundation. February 9, 2025.
8. Wikipedia Contributors. 2025. "Robert Lim." Wikipedia. Wikimedia Foundation. February 17, 2025.

9. Zhang, Fang. 2019. "A Pioneer of Modern Chinese Physiology: Dr. Robert Kho-Seng Lim." Protein & Cell, September. https://doi.org/10.1007/s13238-019-00655-z.

Operations and Advancements

1. "History." 2025. Army.mil. 2025. https://achh.army.mil/history/book-wwii-actvssurgconvol2-chapter14.
2. "History." 2025. Army.mil. 2025. https://achh.army.mil/history/corps-dental-wwii-chapterviii-wwii.
3. Brazelton, M.A. The Production of Penicillin in Wartime China and Sino-American Definitions of "Normal" Microbiology. Retrieved February 19, 2025 fromchrome-extension://efaidnbmnnnibpcajpcglclefindmkaj/https://typeset.io/pdf/the-production-of-penicillin-in-wartime-china-and-sino-3q9sruyzl9.pdf
4. Brazelton, Mary Augusta. 2019. "Engineering Health: Technologies of Immunization in China's Wartime Hinterland, 1937-45." Technology and Culture 60 (2): 409-37. https://doi.org/10.1353/tech.2019.0030.
5. Liu, Michael Shiyung. 2014. "Epidemic Control and Wars in Republican China (1935-1955)." Extrême-Orient, Extrême-Occident, no. 37 (September): 111-39. https://doi.org/10.4000/extremeorient.335.
6. Liu, Michael Shiyung. 2020. "4. Eating Well for Survival: Chinese Nutrition Experiments during World War II." University of Hawaii Press eBooks, February, 89-108. https://doi.org/10.1515/9780824879570-006.
7. Mamlok, Robert. 2018. *The International Medical Relief Corps in Wartime China, 1937-1945*. McFarland.
8. SOON, WAYNE. 2016. "The Wartime Origins of Blood Banking in China, 1943-45." Bulletin of the History of Medicine 90 (3): 424–54. https://doi.org/10.2307/26310928.

Working and Living Conditions

1. "Searching for a Way Forward in China 1944–1945." 2022. Army University Press. 2022. https://www.armyupress.army.mil/Journals/Military-Review/English-Edition-Archives/March-April-2024/Feeding-the-Troops/.
2. 〈中華民國紅十字總會工作概況報告〉（民國 26-28 年）。
3. 《中國紅十字會華北救護委員會報告》。
4. 《抗戰前兩年中之中國紅十字會總會》，頁 5-6。
5. Mamlok, Robert. 2018. *The International Medical Relief Corps in Wartime China, 1937-1945*. McFarland.

國家圖書館出版品預行編目 (CIP) 資料

戰火救援：圖說二戰時期中美醫療合作 = Healing a nation : A photographic history of Sino-American medical collaboration during WWII/Sophia Hu(胡雪慧), Catherine Liu(劉天悅), Angelina Pi(皮妤姍), Ellie Wang(王寶琪) 作；皮妤姍翻譯 . -- 初版 . -- 新北市：喆閎人文工作室, 2025.06
　面；　公分 . -- (歷史影像；3)
中英對照
ISBN 978-626-99335-5-6(平裝)

1.CST: 中國醫學史 2.CST: 國際交流 3.CST: 中美關係 4.CST: 第二次世界大戰

410.92　　　　　　　　　　　　　　114007252

歷史影像 3

戰火救援：圖說二戰時期中美醫療合作
Healing a Nation: A Photographic History of Sino-American Medical Collaboration During WWII

喆閱人文

創 辦 人 / 楊善堯
學術顧問 / 皮國立、林孝庭、劉士永

主編 Edit / 楊善堯 Yang, Shan-Yao
作者 Author / Sophia Hu（胡雪慧）、Catherine Liu（劉天悅）、Angelina Pi（皮妤姍）、
　　　　　　　　Ellie Wang（王寶琪）
翻譯 Translation / 皮妤姍 Angelina Pi
審閱 Proofreading / 陳榮彬 Rong-bin Chen
設計排版 Design Layout / 吳姿穎 Wu, Tzu-Ying
策畫 Collaboration / CompassPoint Mentorship

出版 Publish / 喆閱人文工作室 ZHEHONG HUMANITIES STUDIO
地址 Address / 242011 新北市新莊區中華路一段 100 號 10 樓
　　　　　　　　10F., No. 100, Sec. 1, Zhonghua Rd., Xinzhuang Dist., New Taipei City 242011,
　　　　　　　　Taiwan (R.O.C.)
電話 Telephone / +886-2-2277-0675
信箱 Email / zhehong100101@gmail.com
網站 Website / http://zhehong.tw/
臉書 Facebook / https://www.facebook.com/zhehong10010

初版一刷 First Edition Brush / 2025 年 6 月
定價 Pricing / 新臺幣 NT$ 350 元、美元 USD$ 12 元
ISBN / 978-626-99335-5-6（平裝）
印刷 Print / 秀威資訊科技股份有限公司 Showwe Taiwan

版權所有・翻印必究
All rights reserved. Reproduction will not be tolerated.

如有破損、缺頁或裝訂錯誤，請寄回喆閱人文工作室更換
If there are any damages, missing pages or binding errors,
please send them back to ZHEHONG HUMANITIES STUDIO for replacement.